50 Studies Every Neonatologist Should Know

50 STUDIES EVERY DOCTOR SHOULD KNOW

50 Studies Every Doctor Should Know: The Key Studies that Form the Foundation of Evidence Based Medicine, Revised Edition
Michael E. Hochman

50 Studies Every Internist Should Know
Kristopher Swiger, Joshua R. Thomas, Michael E. Hochman, and Steven Hochman

50 Studies Every Neurologist Should Know
David Y. Hwang and David M. Greer

50 Studies Every Pediatrician Should Know
Ashaunta T. Anderson, Nina L. Shapiro, Stephen C. Aronoff, Jeremiah Davis, and Michael Levy

50 Imaging Studies Every Doctor Should Know
Christoph I. Lee

50 Studies Every Surgeon Should Know
SreyRam Kuy, Rachel J. Kwon, and Miguel A. Burch

50 Studies Every Intensivist Should Know
Edward A. Bittner

50 Studies Every Palliative Care Doctor Should Know
David Hui, Akhila Reddy, and Eduardo Bruera

50 Studies Every Psychiatrist Should Know
Ish P. Bhalla, Rajesh R. Tampi, and Vinod H. Srihari

50 Studies Every Anesthesiologist Should Know
Anita Gupta, Michael E. Hochman, Elena N. Gutman

50 Studies Every Ophthalmologist Should Know
Alan D. Penman, Kimberly W. Crowder, and William M. Watkins, Jr.

50 Studies Every Urologist Should Know
Philipp Dahm

50 Studies Every Obstetrician and Gynecologist Should Know
Constance Liu, Noah Rindos, and Scott Shainker

50 Studies Every Doctor Should Know: The Key Studies that Form the Foundation of Evidence-Based Medicine 2nd Edition
Michael E. Hochman and Steven D. Hochman

50 Studies Every Neonatologist Should Know

EDITED BY

Susanne Hay, MD
Instructor in Pediatrics
Harvard Medical School
Department of Neonatology
Beth Israel Deaconess Medical Center
Boston, MA, USA

Roger F. Soll, MD
H. Wallace Professor of Neonatology
Department of Pediatrics
Larner College of Medicine, University of
Vermont
Director, Vermont Oxford Institute of
Evidence-Based Medicine
Coordinating Editor, Cochrane Neonatal
Burlington, VT, USA

Barbara Schmidt, MD, MSc
Professor, Department of Health Research
Methods, Evidence, and Impact
McMaster University
Hamilton, Ontario, Canada
Professor Emeritus, Department of Pediatrics,
Perelman School of Medicine
University of Pennsylvania
Philadelphia, PA, USA

Haresh Kirpalani, MD, MSc
Professor Emeritus, Department of Pediatrics
The Children's Hospital of Philadelphia,
University Pennsylvania
Philadelphia, PA, USA
Professor Emeritus, Department of Pediatrics
McMaster University
Hamilton, Ontario, Canada

John Zupancic, MD, ScD
Associate Professor of Pediatrics
Harvard Medical School
Associate Chief of Neonatology
Beth Israel Deaconess Medical Center
Boston, MA, USA

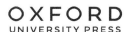

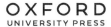

Oxford University Press is a department of the University of Oxford. It furthers
the University's objective of excellence in research, scholarship, and education
by publishing worldwide. Oxford is a registered trade mark of Oxford University
Press in the UK and certain other countries.

Published in the United States of America by Oxford University Press
198 Madison Avenue, New York, NY 10016, United States of America.

Library of Congress Cataloging-in-Publication Data
Names: Hay, Susanne, editor. | Soll, Roger F., editor. | Schmidt, Barbara
  (Barbara K.), editor. | Kirpalani, Haresh, editor. | Zupancic, John, editor.
Title: 50 studies every neonatologist should know / [edited by] Susanne
  Hay, Roger F. Soll, Barbara Schmidt, Haresh Kirpalani, John Zupancic.
Other titles: Fifty studies every neonatologist should know | 50 studies
  every doctor should know (Series)
Description: New York, NY : Oxford University Press, [2024] | Series: Fifty
  studies every doctor should know | Includes bibliographical references
  and index.
Identifiers: LCCN 2024009491 (print) | LCCN 2024009492 (ebook) |
  ISBN 9780197646953 (paperback) | ISBN 9780197646977 (epub) |
  ISBN 9780197646984
Subjects: MESH: Infant, Newborn, Diseases | Neonatology—methods | Infant, Premature
Classification: LCC RJ254 (print) | LCC RJ254 (ebook) | NLM WS 421 |
  DDC 618.92/01—dc23/eng/20240327
LC record available at https://lccn.loc.gov/2024009491
LC ebook record available at https://lccn.loc.gov/2024009492

DOI: 10.1093/med/9780197646953.001.0001

Printed by Marquis Book Printing, Canada

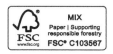

To Jon, Calvin, Elyse, & Juliette—the best things that ever happened to me.

To JZ, my friend and mentor in everything that matters.

And, to Roger, Barbara, and Haresh, who continue to inspire us all.

—Susanne Hay

CONTENTS

Cardiovascular

Respiratory

Nutrition

Thermal

Infectious Disease / Immunology

Hematology

Ophthalmology

Neurology

Intrapartum Care

Health Services

PREFACE FROM THE SERIES EDITOR

When I was a third-year medical student, I asked one of my senior residents—
who seemed to be able to quote every medical study in the history of mankind—
if he had a list of key studies that have defined the current practice of general
medicine which I should read before graduating medical school. "Don't worry,"
he told me. "You will learn the key studies as you go along."

But picking up on these key studies didn't prove so easy, and I was frequently
admonished by my attendings for being unaware of crucial literature in their field.
More importantly, because I had a mediocre understanding of the medical literature, I lacked confidence in my clinical decision-making and had difficulty appre-
ciating the significance of new research findings. It wasn't until I was well into
my residency—thanks to a considerable amount of effort and struggle—that I finally began to feel comfortable with both the emerging and fundamental medical
literature.

Now, as a practicing general internist, I realize that I am not the only doctor
who has struggled to become familiar with the key medical studies that form the
foundation of evidence-based practice. Many of the students and residents I work
with tell me that they feel overwhelmed by the medical literature, and that they
cannot process new research findings because they lack a solid understanding of
what has already been published. Even many practicing physicians—including
those with years of experience—have only a cursory knowledge of the medical
evidence base and make clinical decisions largely on personal experience.

I initially wrote *50 Studies Every Doctor Should Know* in an attempt to provide medical professionals (and even lay readers interested in learning more
about medical research) a quick way to get up to speed on the classic studies
that shape clinical practice. But it soon became clear there was a greater need for
this distillation of the medical evidence than my original book provided. Soon
after the book's publication, I began receiving calls from specialist physicians
in a variety of disciplines wondering about the possibility of another book

focusing on studies in their field. In partnership with a wonderful team of editors from Oxford University Press, we have developed my initial book into a series, offering volumes in Internal Medicine, Pediatrics, Surgery, Neurology, Radiology, Critical Care, Anesthesia, Psychiatry, Palliative Care, Ophthalmology, Urology, Obstetrics and Gynecology, Orthopedics, Global Health, Occupational Therapy, Vascular Surgery—and now Neonatology. Several additional volumes are in the works.

I am particularly excited about this latest volume in Neonatology, which is the culmination of hard work by a team of editors—Susanne Hay, Roger Soll, Barbara Schmidt, Haresh Kirpalani, and John Zupancic—who have summarized the most important studies in their field. Particularly over the past several years, there has become a solid evidence base in the field of Neonatology, and Drs. Hay, Soll, Schmidt, Kirpalani, and Zupancic have effectively captured it in this volume. I believe *50 Studies Every Neonatologist Should Know* provides the perfect launching ground for trainees in the field as well as a helpful refresher for practicing clinicians—physicians, nurse practitioners, and other children's health professionals. The book also highlights key knowledge gaps that may stimulate researchers to tackle key unanswered questions in the field. A special thanks also goes to the wonderful editors at Oxford University Press—Marta Moldvai and Chioma Anomnachi—who injected energy and creativity into the production process for this volume. This volume was a pleasure to help develop, and I learned a lot about the field of Neonatology in the process.

I have no doubt you will gain important insights into the field of Neonatology in the pages ahead!

                                                    Michael E. Hochman, MD, MPH

PREFACE

Neonatology has grown from displaying infants in incubators at carnival sideshows into a sophisticated science that has altered the lives of millions of newborns worldwide. In this book, we attempt to present a snapshot of this scientific evolution, describing a broad range of trials, over time and across topics. As a relatively new field of medicine, neonatology approached the problems of critically ill newborns with energy, invention, and compassion. However, do we know that today's experimental "innovation" will lead to meaningful improvement in outcomes for infants? Dr. Bill Silverman, deemed by many as the "father of neonatal care," showed us how to respond to that challenge. His studies and writings placed our field on strong foundations by encouraging the use and conduct of randomized controlled trials (RCTs). Now, as methods grow more sophisticated, traditional RCTs are joined by other study designs, including cluster, non-inferiority, and adaptive RCTs, all of which are included in this book. Moreover, an evolving appreciation of the importance of bias, evidence quality, and family perspectives/ethics has moved trials forward with improved clarity and clinical impact.

The task of choosing only 50 seminal trials in neonatology was daunting because we faced an embarrassment of riches. In selecting the trials, we have tried to not only illustrate the exceptional history, but also highlight frontiers in their methodology. In addition, we wanted to ensure that various aspects of neonatal care were represented and that there were important learning points in several dimensions. We have consciously been critical, but not with the intention to diminish these contributions to our field. If we are to build a solid future trial environment, we must see where the prior trials succeeded but also where they could have been better. In the following chapters we explore themes including trial design, considerations of bias, implications of early trial termination, issues and limitations of consent, outcome choice and considerations for secondary outcomes, dissemination and adoption, and many others.

In addition to summaries and reviews of the trials, each chapter includes a "Conversation With the Trialist." Trials do not stand alone, and the neonatal community responds to their publication. In order to give the flavor of the type of conversation we argue should take place after a trial is published, we pursued brief interviews with trial authors on one or two salient issues. When the trialists were not available, we added a brief commentary ("A Few Words From the Editor") in place of this section, admittedly substituting our own subjective views. We hope that these pieces still add a useful dimension to the discussion.

Although the extant RCT literature addresses many of our questions in neonatology, not all important aspects, nor all important trials, could be included. Important absences from these chapters include trials of interventions to overcome racial disparities and social determinants of health. We hope that readers of this book will help contribute to the appearance of such studies in our rapidly expanding literature, for the next edition of this book.

Susanne Hay, MD
Roger F. Soll, MD
Barbara Schmidt, MD, MSc
Haresh Kirpalani, MD, MSc
John Zupancic, MD, ScD

CONTRIBUTORS

Elizabeth Baker, PhD
Department of Obstetrics and
    Gynaecology
University of Melbourne
Melbourne, Victoria, Australia

Dirk Bassler, MD
Prof. Dr. med., MSc
Department of Neonatology
University Hospital Zurich, University
    of Zurich
Zurich, Switzerland

**Anna E. Curley, MB MA MD
MRCPI LLB**
Neonatal Consultant, Department of
    Neonatology
National Maternity Hospital
Associate Professor, School
    of Medicine, University
    College Dublin
Dublin, Ireland

Peter G. Davis MBBS, MD
Professor
Newborn Research
The Royal Women's Hospital, The
    University of Melbourne
Melbourne, Victoria, Australia

Sara B. DeMauro, MD MSCE
Associate Professor
Department of Pediatrics
University of Pennsylvania
Philadelphia, PA, USA

Jon Dorling, MBChB, MD
Neonatologist and Honorary
    Professor
Department of Neonatology
Princess Anne Hospital
University Hospital Southampton
Southampton, United Kingdom

Danielle E. Y. Ehret, MD, MPH
Associate Professor of Pediatrics,
    Asfaw Yemiru Green and Gold
    Professor of Global Health
Department of Pediatrics
University of Vermont, Larner College
    of Medicine
Burlington, Vermont, USA

Nicholas D. Embleton, MD
Professor of Neonatal Medicine
Population Health Sciences Institute
Newcastle University
Newcastle upon Tyne, United
    Kingdom

Michelle Fernandes,
MRCPCH DPhil
Academic Clinical Lecturer & MRC
    Clinical Research Training Fellow
    in Paediatrics
MRC Lifecourse Epidemiology
    Centre & Human Development
    and Health Academic Unit, Faculty
    of Medicine
University of Southampton
Southampton, Hampshire, UK
Honorary Senior Research Fellow;
    Nuffield Department of Women's &
    Reproductive Health
Level 3 Women's Centre; John
    Radcliffe Hospital
Associate Fellow; Oxford Maternal
    and Perinatal Health Institute,
    Green Templeton College
University of Oxford
Oxford, Oxfordshire, UK

Elizabeth Foglia, MD MSCE
Associate Professor of Pediatrics
Division of Neonatology, Department
    of Pediatrics
Children's Hospital of Philadelphia
Philadelphia PA, USA

Peter W. Fowlie, MB ChB, FRACP
Consultant Paediatrician
Department of Paediatrics
Dunedin Public Hospital
Dunedin, Otago, New Zealand
Te Whatu Ora (Health New Zealand)

Axel R. Franz, MD
Associated Professor
Neonatology and Center for Pediatric
    Clinical Studies
University Hospital Tübingen
Tübingen, Germany

Christopher Gale, PhD
Professor of Neonatal Medicine
School of Public Health, Faculty of
    Medicine
Imperial College London
London, UK

James I. Hagadorn, MD MSc
Professor of Pediatrics
Division of Neonatology
University of Connecticut School of
    Medicine
Attending Neonatologist
Connecticut Children's
    Medical Center
Hartford, Connecticut, USA

Susanne Hay, MD
Instructor in Pediatrics
Harvard Medical School
Department of Neonatology
Beth Israel Deaconess Medical Center
Boston, Massachusetts, USA

Erik A. Jensen, MD, MSCE
Assistant Professor of Pediatrics
Children's Hospital of Philadelphia
University of Pennsylvania
Philadelphia, Pennsylvania, USA

Stefan Johansson, MD PhD
Associate Professor
Division of Clinical
    Epidemiology, MedS
Karolinska Institutet
Stockholm, Sweden

Anup Katheria, MD
Associate Professor
Department of Neonatology
Sharp Mary Birch Hospital for
    Women & Newborns
San Diego, California, USA

Ashraf Kharrat, MD
MSc(HQ) FRCPC
Assistant Professor
Department of Paediatrics
University of Toronto
Toronto, Ontario, Canada

Seh Hyun Kim, MD
Clinical Professor
Pediatrics
Seoul National University Children's
    Hospital, Seoul National University
    College of Medicine
Seoul, Republic of Korea

Han-Suk Kim, MD, Ph.D.
Professor
Department of Pediatrics
Seoul National University College
    of Medicine/Seoul National
    University Children's Hospital
Jongro, Seoul, Republic of Korea

Brian Christopher King, MD
Assistant Professor
Department of Pediatrics
University of Pittsburgh
Pittsburgh, Pennsylvania, USA

Brianna Liberio, MD
Assistant Professor of Clinical
    Pediatrics
Department of Pediatrics
Indiana University School of
    Medicine
Indianapolis, IN, United States

Li Ma, MD
Associate Professor
Department of Neonatology
Children's Hospital of Hebei
    Province
Shijiazhuang, Hebei, China

Brett J. Manley, MB BS
(Hons), PhD
Associate Professor
Newborn Research
The Royal Women's Hospital
Melbourne, Victoria, Australia

Sarah D. McDonald, MD,
FRCSC, MSc
Professor
Division of Maternal-Fetal Medicine,
    Departments of Obstetrics &
    Gynecology, Radiology & Health
    Research Methods, Evidence
    & Impact
McMaster University
Hamilton, Ontario, Canada

William McGuire, MD
Professor of Child Health
Centre for Reviews and
    Dissemination
University of York
York, United Kingdom

Souvik Mitra, MD PhD FRCPC
Associate Professor
Department of Pediatrics
The University of British Columbia
BC Children's Hospital Research
    Institute
Vancouver, Canada

Adel Mohamed, MD, MSc (Peds),
GDCE (Clin Epi)
Associate Professor, Division of
    Neonatology, University
    of Toronto
Staff Neonatologist, Department of
    Pediatrics, Mount Sinai Hospital
Joseph and Wolf Lebovic Health
    Complex
Toronto, Ontario, Canada

Srinivas Murki, MD, DM
Chief Neonatologist
Department of Neonatology
Paramitha Children Hospital
Hyderabad, Telangana, India

**Evangelia Myttaraki, MD,
MRCPCH, MSc, MM**
Paediatric Trainee
Northwest London Deanery
United Kingdom

**Colm P.F. O'Donnell, MB
FRCPI PhD**
Professor
Neonatal Unit; School of Medicine
National Maternity Hospital;
    University College Dublin
Dublin, Ireland

Wes Onland, MD PhD
Neonatologist
Department of Neonatology
Emma Children's Hospital
    Amsterdam UMC
Amsterdam, The Netherlands

David Osborn, MB BS, MM, PhD
Associate Professor
University of Sydney
Department of Neonatology
Royal Prince Alfred Hospital
Sydney, Australia

Ravi Mangal Patel, MD, MSc
Professor of Pediatrics
Department of Pediatrics
Emory University and Children's
    Healthcare of Atlanta
Atlanta, Georgia, USA

Charles Christoph Roehr, MD PhD
Associate Professor, Clinical Director
Clinical Trials Unit, National Perinatal
    Epidemiology Unit
Oxford Population Health, Medical
    Science Division
University of Oxford
Oxford, UK

Jyotsna Shah, MD
Assistant Professor
Department of Pediatrics
Mount Sinai Hospital
Toronto, Ontario, Canada

Prakesh S. Shah, MD MSc FRCPC
Professor, Department of Pediatrics,
Mount Sinai Hospital and University
    of Toronto
Toronto, Ontario, Canada

M. Jeeva Shankar, MD, DM
Additional Professor
Department of Pediatrics
All India Institute of Medical Sciences
New Delhi, India

Deena Thomas, MD, DM
Consultant Neonatologist
Department of Pediatrics
MGM Muthoot Hospital
Kozhencherry, Kerala, India

Megan J. Turner, MD, MPH
Assistant Professor, University of
    Colorado School of Medicine,
    Department of Pediatrics
Neonatologist, Denver Health
    Medical Center
Denver, Colorado, USA

Anton H. van Kaam, MD, PhD
Professor of Neonatology
Department of Neonatology
Emma Children's Hospital,
    Amsterdam UMC
Amsterdam, The Netherlands

Clyde J. Wright, MD
Professor
Section of Neonatology
Department of Pediatrics
Children's Hospital Colorado and
University of Colorado School of
    Medicine
Aurora, Colorado, USA

John Zupancic, MD, ScD
Associate Professor of Pediatrics
Harvard Medical School
Associate Chief of Neonatology
Beth Israel Deaconess Medical Center
Boston, Massachusetts, USA

ABBREVIATIONS

BPD	bronchopulmonary dysplasia
CA	corrected age
CI	confidence interval
HIE	hypoxic ischemic encephalopathy
IVH	intraventricular hemorrhage
NEC	necrotizing enterocolitis
NICU	neonatal intensive care unit
PDA	patent ductus arteriosus
PMA	postmenstrual age
RCT	randomized controlled trial
ROP	retinopathy of prematurity
RR	relative risk

Additional Notes

Denotation of weeks' gestation is by completed weeks and inclusive when used as a range (e.g., 24 to 27 weeks' = 24 0/7 weeks' to 27 6/7 weeks').

In the Study Overview section, RCTs are masked unless otherwise noted.

Resuscitation

Resuscitation of Asphyxiated Newborn Infants With Room Air or Oxygen

The Resair 2 Trial

PETER G. DAVIS AND ELIZABETH BAKER

"Room air–resuscitated infants . . . recover more quickly than do infants resuscitated with 100% oxygen, as assessed by Apgar scores, time to first breath, and time to first cry."
—SAUGSTAD ET AL.[1]

Research Question: Among asphyxiated newborns with birth weight >999g, does positive pressure ventilation (PPV) using 21% oxygen, compared with 100% oxygen, reduce the combined outcome of death within 7 days and/or moderate or severe hypoxic ischemic encephalopathy (HIE)?

Why Was This Study Done: Resuscitation with 100% oxygen was the long-held standard of care, but with minimal scientific basis and without human studies.

Year Study Began: 1994

Year Study Published: 1998

Study Location: India, Egypt, Philippines, Estonia, Spain, Norway (11 centers total)

Who Was Studied: Infants with birth weight >999g who received PPV at birth because they were either (i) apneic or (ii) gasping with a heart rate <80 beats per minute (bpm)

Who Was Excluded: Infants with lethal anomalies, hydrops, or cyanotic congenital heart defects; and stillbirths

How Many Patients: 703. An initial sample size of 920 was proposed.

Study Overview: Resair (RESuscitation of asphyxiated newborn infants with room AIR) 2 was a parallel-group, unmasked, quasi-randomized trial (Figure 1.1).

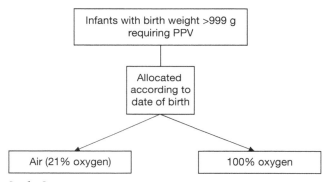

Figure 1.1 Study Overview

What Were the Interventions:
- Infants allocated to the air group received PPV with 21% oxygen. If heart rates remained <80 bpm or central cyanosis was present within 90 seconds, infants were switched to 100% oxygen.
- Infants randomized to the 100% oxygen group received PPV with 100% oxygen.

How Long Was Follow-up: 28 days

What Were the Endpoints:
Primary outcome: Composite outcome of death within one week or moderate/severe HIE.
Selected secondary outcomes: 5-minute Apgar score, time to first breath/cry, duration of resuscitation, death at 28 days.

Concerns Regarding Bias: This study was at high risk of allocation, selection, and performance/detection biases; given the quasi-randomized design (alternate-day allocation by date of birth) and the lack of masking of caregivers to the intervention.

RESULTS

- The composite outcome of death in the first 7 days or moderate/severe HIE did not differ between the 21% oxygen group (21.2%) and the 100% oxygen group (23.7%) (odds ratio 0.94, 95% confidence interval [CI] 0.63 to 1.40).
- There were no differences in the components of the primary outcome, and no difference in mortality rates at 28 days.
- Some early markers of HIE were better in infants managed in air compared with 100% oxygen. These included fewer infants with 5-minute Apgar scores <7 ($p = 0.030$) and shorter times to first breath and first cry ($p = 0.004$ and 0.006, respectively).
- There were no significant differences in 10-minute Apgar scores, heart rate, or oxygen saturations in the first 30 minutes, or duration of resuscitation.

Criticisms and Limitations: The delivery room is a challenging setting for any clinical trial. It is very difficult to gain prospective consent; the environment is stressful; and events are fast-moving. Gold standard design features like randomization and blinding of the intervention, while adding to the certainty of the evidence derived from a study, make it considerably more difficult to perform. Few trials of interventions in the delivery room had been conducted to this point, and there was only one small, single center trial on the topic of oxygen concentrations for neonatal resuscitation.[2] There was a marked lack of equipoise regarding this question. The conventional wisdom of the time was, "Oxygen is vital, not just useful. One breath of oxygen is worth 5 breaths of air in this situation."[3] Notwithstanding design issues, completing a large, international trial under those circumstances was a remarkable achievement.

Other Relevant Studies and Information:
- Systematic reviews performed since Resair 2 have confirmed that resuscitation of term infants with 21% oxygen results in lower mortality rates than 100% oxygen.[4-6] The most recent, performed by the International Liaison Committee on Resuscitation (ILCOR) Neonatal Life Support Task Force, included 5 randomized controlled trials and

5 quasi-randomized trials, and demonstrated a reduction in short-term mortality for term infants resuscitated with air (relative risk 0.73, 95% CI 0.57 to 0.94).
- Follow-up at 18 to 24 months of infants enrolled in Resair 2 was reported separately and showed no significant differences in growth parameters or rates of neurologic impairment.[7]
- In 2020, ILCOR stated, "for newborn infants at 35 weeks' or greater gestation receiving respiratory support at birth, we suggest starting with 21% oxygen."[8]

Summary and Implications: Resair 2 made several important contributions to neonatal medicine. First, it demonstrated that it was possible to allocate newborn infants to 2 different resuscitation strategies in the seconds following birth in an international, multicentered trial. It facilitated further studies to answer this question which were performed to higher methodological standards. It also provided a template to address other important questions to fill the evidence vacuum of delivery room care. Finally, the findings themselves, in combination with studies that followed, led to an important practice change saving countless lives around the world.

A CONVERSATION WITH THE TRIALIST: OLA SAUGSTAD

What gave you the courage to challenge the long-standing practice of resuscitation with 100% oxygen?

The idea to supplement pure oxygen to asphyxiated babies was deeply rooted in the tradition, although the idea had never been tested out scientifically.

[From studies in the 1970s, we concluded] that the combination of a high hypoxanthine level with high oxygen concentration, which was the case during resuscitation, might be detrimental.

In 1992, we described a newborn hypoxic piglet model with similar/identical recovery [when] either 100% oxygen or air was applied during the resuscitation. The year after we published our pilot study from India together with Siddarth Ramji's team in New Delhi indicating use of air is safe. In 1998, we consequently published Resair 2, a multicenter study showing a strong tendency to reduced mortality in asphyxic newborn infants ventilated with air compared to 100% Oxygen. Although WHO recommended air already in 1998 . . . it took another 12 years before ILCOR changed their guidelines from recommending 100% oxygen to air.

What did you learn about combining sites from high-income areas with low-income areas?

The difference in mortality was extremely high, making it challenging to lump all results together. Especially in the USA our data were not considered relevant because most of them were collected in low-income countries. Today we would have carried out separate studies in high- and low-income areas, and in fact, there are now several such studies from each category.

What else do we need to know about oxygen for resuscitation of term infants?

There are still subgroups of newborn babies, such as babies with some congenital malformations, or babies needing chest compressions, in which we don't know the optimal initial oxygen concentration during resuscitation.

References

1. Saugstad OD, Rootwelt T, Aalen O. Resuscitation of asphyxiated newborn infants with room air or oxygen: an international controlled trial: the Resair 2 study. *Pediatrics.* 1998;102(1):e1.
2. Ramji S, Ahuja S, Thirupuram S, et al. Resuscitation of asphyxic newborn infants with room air or 100% oxygen. *Pediatr Res.* 1993;34(6):809–12.
3. Ainley-Walker JC. Resuscitation of the newborn. *Br Med J.* 1979;2(6204):1590.
4. Davis PG, Tan A, O'Donnell CP, et al. Resuscitation of newborn infants with 100% oxygen or air: a systematic review and meta-analysis. *Lancet.* 2004;364(9442):1329–33.
5. Saugstad OD, Ramji S, Vento M. Resuscitation of depressed newborn infants with ambient air or pure oxygen: a meta-analysis. *Biol Neonate.* 2005;87(1):27–34.
6. Welsford M, Nishiyama C, Shortt C, et al. Room air for initiating term newborn resuscitation: a systematic review with meta-analysis. *Pediatrics.* 2019;143(1):e20181825.
7. Saugstad OD, Ramji S, Irani SF, et al. Resuscitation of newborn infants with 21% or 100% oxygen: follow-up at 18 to 24 months. *Pediatrics.* 2003;112(2):296–300.
8. Wyckoff MH, Wyllie J, Aziz K, et al. Neonatal Life Support: 2020 International Consensus on Cardiopulmonary Resuscitation and Emergency Cardiovascular Care Science With Treatment Recommendations. *Circulation.* 2020;142(16_suppl_1):S185–s221.

2

Delivery Room Management of the Apparently Vigorous Meconium-Stained Neonate

CHARLES CHRISTOPH ROEHR

"In this trial, we found routine suctioning of the apparently vigorous meconium-stained infant to be no better than expectant management in preventing MAS or other respiratory disorders."

—WISWELL ET AL.[1]

Research Question: In vigorous newborn infants born through meconium-stained amniotic fluid (MSAF), does intubation and tracheal suctioning, as compared with expectant management, reduce the incidence of meconium aspiration syndrome (MAS)?

Why Was This Study Done: Intubation and tracheal suctioning were recommended for vigorous infants born through MSAF, based on observational reports. At the time of this study, there was conflicting evidence for a more selective approach to intubation and suctioning, without strong RCT data.

Year Study Began: 1995

Year Study Published: 2000

Study Location: United States, Argentina, Paraguay (12 centers total)

Who Was Studied: Vigorous newborn term infants born through MSAF

Who Was Excluded: Infants born through MSAF who were declared "non-vigorous" (lack of tone, no respiratory effort, heart rate below 100 beats per minute) at birth

How Many Patients: 2094

Study Overview: This was a parallel-group, unmasked RCT (Figure 2.1).

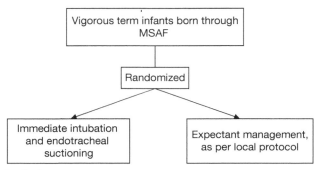

Figure 2.1 Study Overview

What Were the Interventions:
- Infants randomized to immediate intubation and suctioning were intubated immediately after birth, following assessment for vigor. They received tracheal suctioning, repeated until no additional MSAF could be retrieved. This was followed by immediate extubation.
- Infants randomized to expectant management received routine delivery room care and monitoring as per the local unit's protocols.

How Long Was Follow-up: Hospital discharge

What Were the Endpoints:
Primary outcome: MAS, defined as "respiratory distress in an infant born through MSAF whose symptoms could not be otherwise explained."
Selected secondary outcomes: Other respiratory disorders, complications of intubation procedure.

Concerns Regarding Bias: The study was at high risk for performance/detection bias, as caregivers were not blinded to the intervention. Additional bias may be present, as 89% of studied infants were from 6 of 12 centers. However, outcomes were similar across centers (unpublished data; see A Conversation With the Trialist).

RESULTS

- Routine suctioning of the apparently vigorous infant born through MSAF was no better than expectant management in preventing MAS (3.2% versus 2.7%) or other respiratory disorders (3.8% versus 4.5%). Even with the thickest consistency MSAF, intratracheal suctioning was no better than expectant management in preventing respiratory illness.
- Complications of intubation procedures were infrequent (complication rate 3.8%), not related to operator seniority, and mostly transient.
- Risk factors for respiratory disorders following birth through MSAF included: delivery by Caesarean section, Apgar score <6 at 1 or 5 minutes, oligohydramnios, lack of fetal heart rate (FHR) monitoring and abnormal FHR monitoring, thickness of meconium at birth, not having oropharyngeal suctioning performed at birth, and <5 antenatal visits.

Criticisms and Limitations: This was the largest RCT to investigate the management of vigorous meconium-stained infants.[2] At the time, management included suctioning at the perineum and intubation and suctioning of all meconium-stained infants, whether vigorous or not. This trial continued with the immediate postpartum suctioning of the oropharynx but addressed only the vigorous infants. The authors obtained a waiver of consent. The rationale for this included the emergent nature of MSAF, the inherent difficulties in obtaining valid informed consent from a mother undergoing the pain of labor, the lack of generalizability inherent to individual consent in an emergent situation,[3] and the efficiency of trial enrollment. To ensure ethical practice, Wiswell et al. sought extensive advice from parent representatives and ethicists and had the explicit support from national pediatric societies and the trial funders. Moreover, individual Institutional Review Board review was obtained at most study centers. Nonetheless, a present-day trial ethical board review would very likely demand at minimum waivers or deferral of consent.[4]

Since this study, proficiency in endotracheal intubation among the pediatric workforce has decreased. This reflects several changes in neonatal airway management, including the more frequent expectant management of infants born through MSAF.[5]

Other Relevant Studies and Information:
- Subsequent studies further defined the role of suctioning on the perineum and endotracheal intubation of non-vigorous infants.
- Trials of oropharyngeal and nasopharyngeal suctioning of meconium-stained neonates before delivery of their shoulders demonstrated no difference in MAS (4% versus 4%; RR 0.9, 95% CI 0.6 to 1.3).[6] A systematic review identified 8 RCTs, including >4000 infants, and reported no differences in mortality or need for resuscitation for hypoxic ischemic encephalopathy.[7]
- With regard to non-vigorous infants born through MSAF, the evidence for tracheal suctioning on the incidence of MAS and its complications is limited.[8]
- In 2015, the International Liaison Committee on Resuscitation (ILCOR) formally recommended against the routine practice of intubation of all (vigorous and non-vigorous) infants born though MSAF.[9] However, subsequent observational studies reported concerning neonatal outcomes in non-vigorous infants after such protocol changes.[10,11] A recent systematic review of studies investigating the routine versus "as indicated" tracheal suctioning of non-vigorous babies born through MSAF highlighted the overall low certainty of evidence, limiting strong recommendations for or against routine tracheal suctioning.[12]

Summary and Implications: Wiswell et al. showed that vigorous term infants born through MSAF can be successfully managed with expectant management, rather than routine intubation and endotracheal suctioning. This trial led practice change away from routine intubation and paved the way towards supportive, noninvasive management for infants born through MSAF, although questions remain regarding management of the non-vigorous infant.

A CONVERSATION WITH THE TRIALIST: DR. THOMAS E. WISWELL

How, in your view, has your study contributed to the review of the consent process for studies in the delivery room?

More than 20 years after publication of this investigation, there are still a number of interventions routinely performed on neonates in the delivery room, interventions that have not undergone comprehensive evaluation of their effectiveness by the gold standard: a well-designed, appropriately powered randomized, controlled trial

(RCT). As we describe in the discussion section of the publication, due to inherent difficulties in obtaining informed consent in the delivery room or other emergency situations, a large proportion of the patient population that may need an intervention would not be enrolled into such an RCT if preceding informed consent were mandatory. For a trial in which 30%–40% or more of the eligible population cannot be enrolled, the results would be questionable. In order to find an evidence-based "answer" as to whether or not a widely practiced, unproven intervention in emergency situations is appropriate, a waiver of consent may be needed.

A range of recruitment is represented among the included centers. How confident can we be that results from less actively recruiting units are similar to larger recruiting sites?

Approximately 90% of the study infants were born in the 6 sites that each enrolled 197–408 subjects. The various outcomes were similar among these sites, as well as in the total of 227 infants born in the remaining 6 lower-recruiting sites (unpublished data that was assessed during analysis). Hence, we are very confident about the results.

References

1. Wiswell TE, Gannon CM, Jacob J, et al. Delivery room management of the apparently vigorous meconium-stained neonate: results of the multicenter, international collaborative trial. *Pediatrics.* 2000;105:1–7.
2. Halliday HL, Sweet DG. Endotracheal intubation at birth for preventing morbidity and mortality in vigorous, meconium-stained infants born at term. *Cochrane Database Syst Rev.* 2001;(1):CD000500.
3. Songstad NT, Roberts CT, Manley BJ, et al. Retrospective consent in a neonatal randomized controlled trial. *Pediatrics.* 2018;141:e20172092.
4. Rich WD, Katheria AC. Waived consent in perinatal/neonatal research-when is it appropriate? *Front Pediatr.* 2019 Nov 26;7:493.
5. Belkhatir K, Scrivens A, O'Shea JE, et al. Experience and training in endotracheal intubation and laryngeal mask airway use in neonates: results of a national survey. *Arch Dis Child Fetal Neonatal Ed.* 2021;106:223–24.
6. Vain NE, Szyld EG, Prudent LM, et al. Oropharyngeal and nasopharyngeal suctioning of meconium-stained neonates before delivery of their shoulders: multicentre, randomised controlled trial. *Lancet.* 2004;364:597–602.
7. Foster JP, Dawson JA, Davis PG, et al. Routine oro/nasopharyngeal suction versus no suction at birth. *Cochrane Database Syst Rev.* 2017;4(4):CD010332.
8. Nangia S, Thukral A, Chawla D. Tracheal suction at birth in non-vigorous neonates born through meconium-stained amniotic fluid. *Cochrane Database Syst Rev.* 2021;6(6):CD012671.
9. Perlman JM, Wyllie J, Kattwinkel J, et al.; Neonatal Resuscitation Chapter Collaborators. Part 7: Neonatal Resuscitation: 2015 International Consensus on

Cardiopulmonary Resuscitation and Emergency Cardiovascular Care Science With Treatment Recommendations (Reprint). *Pediatrics*. 2015;136 Suppl 2:S120–66.

10. Chiruvolu A, Miklis KK, Chen E, et al. Delivery room management of meconium-stained newborns and respiratory support. *Pediatrics*. 2018;142:e20181485.

11. Kalra V, Leegwater AJ, Vadlaputi P, et al. Neonatal outcomes of non-vigorous neonates with meconium-stained amniotic fluid before and after change in tracheal suctioning recommendation. *J Perinatol*. 2022;42:769–74.

12. Ramaswamy VV, Bandyopadhyay T, Nangia S, et al. Assessment of change in practice of routine tracheal suctioning approach of non-vigorous infants born through meconium-stained amniotic fluid: a pragmatic systematic review and meta-analysis of evidence outside randomized trials. *Neonatology*. 2023;120:161–75.

3

Randomized Trial of Occlusive Wrap for Heat Loss Prevention in Preterm Infants

The HeLP Trial

ANUP KATHERIA

"Because this study was not powered to detect a difference in mortality within strata, we cannot be sure that there is no lifesaving benefit accrued by wrapping infants born at less than 25 6/7 weeks' gestation."
—REILLY ET AL.[1]

Research Question: In extremely preterm infants, does the application of a polyethylene occlusive wrap immediately after delivery, compared with conventional management of drying and thermal management, reduce all-cause mortality before hospital discharge or 6 months' CA?

Why Was This Study Done: Hypothermia is a risk factor for mortality in very immature infants. Occlusive wrap placed on extremely preterm infants after birth can reduce postnatal evaporative heat loss. Two prior small studies by members of this group demonstrated reduced hypothermia and decreased mortality.[2,3] However, results of meta-analysis including other small studies remained inconclusive for the outcome of death.[4]

Year Study Began: 2004

Year Study Published: 2015

Study Location: United States, Canada, Spain, Portugal, Singapore, Ireland, Malaysia (39 centers)

Who Was Studied: Infants between 24 0/7 and 27 6/7 weeks' gestation, with firm decision prior to birth to provide full resuscitation measures.[5]

Who Was Excluded: Infants born with major congenital anomalies not covered by skin (e.g., gastroschisis, meningomyelocele). Infants born with blistering skin conditions that preclude the use of occlusive wrap.[5]

How Many Patients: The study was powered on a sample size of 1604, to demonstrate a 25% relative risk reduction in mortality. However, despite a 10 year duration, the trial was terminated early, with only 817 infants enrolled and 801 analyzed.

Study Overview: The HeLP (Heat Loss Prevention) trial was a parallel-group, unmasked RCT (Figure 3.1). Randomization was stratified by site and by gestational age (24 to 25 weeks and 26 to 27 weeks).

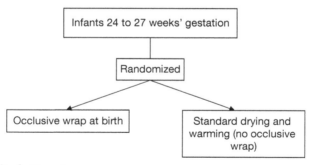

Figure 3.1 Study Overview

What Were the Interventions:
- Patients randomized to the intervention group had a polyethylene occlusive skin wrap applied immediately after birth and removed after the infant has been admitted to a stable thermoneutral environment.
- Patients randomized to the control group received routine care of drying and warming only.

How Long Was Follow-up: Hospital discharge or 6 months' CA, whichever came first.

What Were the Endpoints:
Primary outcome: All-cause mortality.
Selected secondary outcomes: Axillary temperature after stabilization, Apgar scores, and common complications of prematurity (including PDA, pulmonary hemorrhage, and IVH).

Concerns Regarding Bias: The study was at high risk for performance/detection bias, as caregivers were not blinded to the intervention. Additional bias may be present with early termination of study enrollment for futility.

RESULTS

- Rates of death in the 2 groups were similar (20.5% versus 20%; odds ratio [OR] 1.0, 95% CI 0.7 to 1.5, $p = 0.85$), despite a 10 year recruitment period.
- However, there was only a 0.6 degree improvement in the temperature achieved by the intervention.
- Among the secondary outcomes, a lower 1-minute Apgar score was found in the occlusive wrap group, and there was a decrease in pulmonary hemorrhage in the occlusive wrap group.
- In the lower gestational age stratum (24 to 25 weeks' gestation), there was a decrease in the risk of treated PDA and pulmonary hemorrhage in the occlusive wrap group.

Criticisms and Limitations: Early termination of a trial can be problematic, especially for evaluation of secondary and other exploratory outcomes, such as the effect at lower gestational ages. While the trial was not likely to detect the expected 25% relative risk reduction in mortality, it may have been able to look at differences in secondary outcomes in the lower gestational age group with greater statistical power. It is not clear why it took 10 years to recruit this sample. Over that time, concerns on temperature, especially for low birth weight infants, was increasing, and there may have been additional evolutions in practice to prevent this.

There were a high number of protocol violations in correct placement of the occlusive wrap. While the temperatures were still higher than in the no wrap group, this may have reduced the efficacy of the intervention between the groups. Even so, the temperature difference achieved was modest.

The use of antenatal consent for the majority of the study participants may have further limited the generalizability of the trial, since women with threatened extremely preterm birth who can be approached for consent and enrolled may not be representative of the entire population. Only 4 of 39 sites obtained a waiver of antenatal consent for the intervention. Eighty-three percent of the infants were enrolled under informed consent, and 17% were enrolled under a waiver of consent. A recent exploratory analysis by this group demonstrated that infants born at centers requiring antenatal consent were more likely to have mothers who had received the potentially life-saving therapy of antenatal steroids (p <0.0001).[6]

Other Relevant Studies and Information:
- McCall et al. performed a meta-analysis of 25 studies across 15 comparison groups to test interventions to prevent hypothermia compared with routine care applied within 10 minutes of life for preterm infants.[7] They reinforced that plastic wraps or bags reduce hypothermia, but there is limited evidence of improvement in any short-term morbidities including death. They suggest that hypothermia may be a marker for illness severity, rather than a cause for these morbidities.
- A strong birth weight relationship appears to be present in a smaller, earlier trial which achieved a higher temperature in infants <750 g birth weight.[3]
- The 2005 American Academy of Pediatrics guidelines, published while this trial was underway, recommended use of a polyethylene bag as part of a bundle of interventions to prevent hypothermia in preterm infants <1500 g birth weight.[8] Current guidelines continue to support these measures.[9]

Summary and Implications: The HeLP trial confirmed that early occlusive wrap in extremely preterm infants reduces the risk of hypothermia. Indeed, at the time the HeLP trial was performed, many centers had begun to adopt measures to reduce heat loss in extremely preterm infants based on the AAP guidelines published in 2006.[8] Although this large trial reinforced the safety of the use of occlusive wraps and their efficacy in reducing hypothermia, it did not provide any evidence that use of the wrap reduces mortality. Despite the lack of longer term clinical benefits, the results of this trial support the use of occlusive wraps to reduce hypothermia on admission to the NICU. Current international guidelines continue to recommend plastic wrap for delivery room care of very preterm infants.[9]

A FEW WORDS FROM THE EDITOR

The HeLP Trial was undertaken based in part on small trials and the land-mark work of Silverman and colleagues (See Chapter 24 on Silverman's thermal environment trial), which suggested that an improvement in survival seemed plausible. Yet, as is often the case, a larger study did not substantiate the early promise shown in smaller trials.[1] Why is this so often the case? Perhaps the issue is a failure to understand the disease process or mechanism of the intervention, in this case the relationship of hypothermia compared with the more profound differences reported by Silverman. Despite the lack of benefit on mortality, use of occlusive wrap has been widely adopted as an inexpensive and straightforward way to minimize heat loss.

—Roger Soll

1. Ioannidis JPA. Why most discovered true associations are inflated. *Epidemiology.* 2008;19:640–8.

References

1. Reilly MC, Vohra S, Rac VE, et al. Randomized trial of occlusive wrap for heat loss prevention in preterm infants. *J Pediatr.* 2015;166(2):262–8.e2.
2. Vohra V, Frent G, Campbell V, et al. Effect of polyethylene occlusive skin wrapping on heat loss in very low birth weight infants at delivery: a randomized trial. *J Pediatr.* 1999;134(5):547–51.
3. Vohra S, Roberts RS, Zhang B, et al. Heat loss prevention (HeLP) in the delivery room: a randomized controlled trial of polyethylene occlusive skin wrapping in very preterm infants. *J Pediatr.* 2004;145:750–53.
4. Cramer K, Wiebe N, Hartling L, et al. Heat loss prevention: a systematic review of occlusive skin wrap for premature neonates. *J Perinatol.* 2005;25(12):763–9.
5. Vohra S, Reilly M, Rac VE, et al. Study protocol for multicentre randomized controlled trial of HeLP (Heat Loss Prevention) in the delivery room. *Contemp Clin Trials.* 2013;36:54–60.
6. Vohra S, Reilly M, Rac VE. Differences in demographics and outcomes based on method of consent for a randomised controlled trial on heat loss prevention in the delivery room. *Arch Dis Child Fetal Neonatal Ed.* 2021 Mar;106(2):118–24.
7. McCall EM, Alderdice F, Halliday HL, Vohra S, Johnston L. Interventions to prevent hypothermia at birth in preterm and/or low birth weight infants. *Cochrane Database Syst Rev.* 2018;2(2):CD004210.
8. American Heart Association, American Academy of Pediatrics. 2005 American Heart Association (AHA) Guidelines for Cardiopulmonary Resuscitation (CPR) and Emergency Cardiovascular Care (ECC) of Pediatric and Neonatal Patients: Neonatal Resuscitation Guidelines. *Pediatrics.* 2006;117(5):e1029–38.
9. Wyckoff MH, Weiner CGM,; Neonatal Life Support Collaborators. 2020 international consensus on cardiopulmonary resuscitation and emergency cardiovascular care science with treatment recommendations. *Pediatrics* 2021;147:e2020038505C.

4

Association of Umbilical Cord Milking vs Delayed Umbilical Cord Clamping With Death or Severe Intraventricular Hemorrhage Among Preterm Infants

The PREMOD2 Trial

SEH HYUN KIM AND HAN-SUK KIM

"In this post hoc analysis of a prematurely terminated randomized clinical trial of umbilical cord milking versus delayed umbilical cord clamping among preterm infants born at less than 32 weeks' gestation, there was no statistically significant difference in the rate of a composite outcome of death or severe intraventricular hemorrhage, but there was a statistically significantly higher rate of severe intraventricular hemorrhage in the umbilical cord milking group."

—KATHERIA ET AL.[1]

Research Question: Is there a difference in the rate of death or severe IVH in preterm infants delivered at 23 to 31 weeks' gestation receiving placental transfusion from umbilical cord milking (UCM) or delayed cord clamping (DCC)?

Why Was This Study Done: Cord milking had been introduced into practice as an alternative to delayed cord clamping, in hopes of providing the benefit of placental transfusion to preterm infants without delaying resuscitation. However, cord milking remained insufficiently tested.

Year Study Began: 2017

Year Study Published: 2019

Study Location: United States, Germany, Canada, Ireland (9 centers total)

Who Was Studied: Preterm infants delivered between 23 and 31 weeks' gestation

Who Was Excluded: Infants with major congenital anomalies, severe placental abruption, transplacental incision, umbilical cord prolapse, hydrops, bleeding accreta, monochorionic multiple births, other fetal or maternal risk of severe compromise at delivery, or family unlikely to return for 24-month neurodevelopmental testing.

How Many Patients: 474. Of note, this trial was powered for a sample size of 1500, but was ended early for a higher rate of severe IVH in the UCM group on the recommendation of the Data Safety Monitoring Board.

Study Overview: The Premature Infants Receiving Milking or Delayed Cord Clamping (PREMOD2) trial was designed as a non-inferiority, parallel-group, unmasked RCT (Figure 4.1); with randomization stratified by gestational age (<28 weeks, ≥28 weeks).

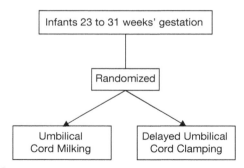

Figure 4.1 Study Overview

What Were the Interventions:
Interventions for both groups were performed with infants held below the level of the cesarean incision or below the level of the introitus for vaginal delivery.

- Patients randomized to the UCM group had the umbilical cord milked by an obstetrician. Approximately 20 cm of the umbilical cord was milked for 2 seconds, allowing refill, and repeated 3 times.
- Patients randomized to the DCC group were wrapped in warm, sterile towels after delivery and held for at least 60 seconds prior to umbilical cord clamping by an obstetrician. To stimulate respiratory effort during this time, infants were dried and given gentle tactile stimulation.

How Long Was Follow-up: 6 months' CA

What Were the Endpoints:
Primary outcome: Composite outcome of death or severe IVH at 6 months' CA.
Selected secondary outcomes: Components of the composite primary outcome, any grade of IVH, hemoglobin and hematocrit levels.

Concerns Regarding Bias: The study was at high risk for performance bias, as parents/caregivers were not blinded to the intervention; however, all outcome assessments were performed by blinded team members. There was risk of additional bias from both the early termination of enrollment and a large number of post-randomization exclusions (66 of 540 infants). Attempts were made to standardize protocols by videotaped assessments of the first trial resuscitation at each site.

RESULTS

- The planned non-inferiority analysis could not be performed because of the early termination of the study.
- In post hoc analysis, there was no statistically significant difference in the rates of the original composite outcome of death or severe IVH between the UCM group and the DCC group (12% versus 8%; Risk Difference [RD] 0.04, 95% CI –0.02 to 0.09, $p = 0.16$).
- UCM was associated with a higher rate of severe IVH than DCC (8% versus 3%; RD 0.05, 95% CI 0.01 to 0.09, $p = 0.02$).
- The concerning risk of severe IVH with UCM was mostly seen in infants delivered at 23 to 27 weeks' gestation.

Criticisms and Limitations: This non-inferiority RCT of preterm infants was terminated early for harm. As discussed in a separate chapter (See Chapter 5 on the SAIL trial.), early termination can lead towards exaggerated effects.[2] As acknowledged by the trial authors, the early termination of their trial precludes any definitive conclusions.

Other Relevant Studies and Information:

- Earlier work from this team demonstrated higher systemic blood flow with UCM as compared with DCC, without meaningful differences in clinical outcomes.[3]
- A Cochrane review performed prior to publication of this trial's results included 14 RCTs (involving 1505 infants) comparing UCM to immediate or delayed cord clamping and concluded that there were no significant benefits or hazards associated with UCM.[4]
- A recent review that included this study found no clear differences for severe IVH, NEC, or hyperbilirubinemia.[5]
- The publication of this trial led the American College of Obstetricians and Gynecologists (ACOG) to recommend against UCM for infants <28 weeks' gestation.[6]
- Planned follow-up analysis of this cohort at 22 to 26 months' CA is underway.[1]

Summary and Implications: The PREMOD2 trial was terminated early for concern about increased risks of severe IVH after cord milking. In their post hoc analysis, the authors found no difference in composite rates of death or severe IVH, but an increase in the rate of severe IVH in preterm infants receiving UCM versus DCC. The trial detected a potentially worrying safety signal for a common clinical practice, discouraging umbilical milking pending further trial evidence.

A CONVERSATION WITH THE TRIALIST: ANUP KATHERIA

What are the inherent advantages of umbilical cord milking (UCM) that led to your initial design of a non-inferiority trial? If the need to immediately resuscitate an infant is seen as an advantage, should studies be limited to infants that either receive UCM or immediate cord clamping?

Our initial pilot study had demonstrated that UCM provided a greater placental transfusion compared to DCC in infants delivered by cesarean section. However, since DCC was still widely practiced it was prudent to design the trial as a non-inferiority study to determine whether UCM was safe and well tolerated by preterm infants in a much larger trial. While a study comparing UCM to immediate cord clamping would be more reasonable, it would be difficult to ethically conduct such a study unless it were conducted in infants that required resuscitation at birth. This is part of the reason why we are conducting a study in term–near term non-vigorous infants using a waivered consent approach. This would be the only method to conduct a study in preterm infants, but unlike term–near term infants who may need immediate assistance at birth due to asphyxia, preterm infants are more likely to initiate breathing on their own if given enough time.

Given the meta-analysis showing no overall harm, do you think there should be a new trial?

A second large trial would be ideal since our study suffers from a risk of a type 2 error, given that it was stopped early for harm. Ideally, a trial that included many extremely preterm infants 23–27 weeks' GA would be able to better validate or refute our findings. Unfortunately, several current and past trials that enroll infants between 23 [and] 32 weeks' GA, often enroll more of the mature infants (average gestational age 28 weeks) limiting the ability to detect any harmful effects of cord milking at the lowest gestation.

We have completed enrollment (N = 1019) in infants 28–32 weeks, and those results should be presented and published this year to support the safety in this population.

References

1. Katheria A, Reister F, Essers J, et al. Association of umbilical cord milking vs delayed umbilical cord clamping with death or severe intraventricular hemorrhage among preterm infants. *JAMA*. 2019;322:1877–86.
2. Guyatt GH, Briel M, Glasziou P, et al. Problems of stopping trials early. *BMJ*. 2012;344:e3863.
3. Katheria AC, Truong G, Cousins L, et al. Umbilical cord milking versus delayed cord clamping in preterm infants. *Pediatrics*. 2015;136(1):61–9.
4. Rabe H, Gyte GM, Diaz-Rossello JL, et al. Effect of timing of umbilical cord clamping and other strategies to influence placental transfusion at preterm birth on maternal and infant outcomes. *Cochrane Database Syst Rev*. 2019;9:CD003248.
5. Seidler AL, Gyte GML, Rabe H, et al. Umbilical cord management for newborns <34 weeks' gestation: a meta-analysis. *Pediatrics*. 2021;147(3):e20200576.
6. Delayed umbilical cord clamping after birth. American College of Obstetricians and Gynecologists. ACOG Committee Opinion No. 814. Washington, DC: American College of Obstetricians and Gynecologists. *Obstet Gynecol*. 2020;136:e100–6.

5

Effect of Sustained Inflations vs Intermittent Positive Pressure Ventilation on Bronchopulmonary Dysplasia or Death Among Extremely Preterm Infants

The SAIL Trial

SUSANNE HAY AND JOHN ZUPANCIC

"These findings do not support the use of ventilation with sustained inflations among extremely preterm infants, although early termination of the trial limits definitive conclusions."

—KIRPALANI ET AL.[1]

Research Question: Among extremely preterm infants requiring resuscitation at birth, does a strategy including sustained inflations (SI), compared with standard intermittent positive pressure ventilation, reduce BPD or death at 36 week's PMA without harm?

Why Was This Study Done: Although animal models seemed to offer strong support for this approach, limited trial evidence on sustained inflation was available prior to this study.[2,3]

Year Study Began: 2014

Year Study Published: 2019

Study Location: United States, Australia, the Netherlands, Canada, Germany, Italy, Austria, South Korea, and Singapore (18 NICUs total)

Who Was Studied: Infants between 23 and 26 weeks' gestation requiring positive pressure resuscitation at birth for inadequate respiratory effort or heart rate <100 beats per minute

Who Was Excluded: Infants deemed nonviable or with major anomalies.

How Many Patients: 460

Study Overview: The SAIL (Sustained Aeration for Infant Lungs) trial was a parallel-group, unmasked RCT (Figure 5.1).

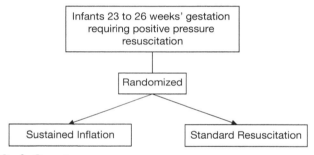

Figure 5.1 Study Overview

What Were the Interventions:
- Patients randomized to the intervention group received a sustained inflation in the immediate neonatal period at a peak pressure of 20 cm H_2O for 15 seconds. If no response in breathing pattern, this was followed by a second sustained inflation at a peak pressure 25 cm H_2O for 15 seconds. Sustained inflations were delivered via a face mask or nasopharyngeal tube attached to a T-piece resuscitator.
- Patients randomized to the control group received routine intermittent positive pressure ventilation with positive end-expiratory pressure.

How Long Was Follow-up: Hospital discharge

What Were the Endpoints:
Primary outcome: Death or BPD at 36 weeks' PMA.
Selected secondary outcomes: Death within 48 hours, pneumothorax, pulmonary interstitial emphysema, respiratory outcomes following delivery.

Concerns Regarding Bias: This study was at high risk for performance/detection bias, as blinding of caregivers to intervention was not possible.

RESULTS

- Of note, trial recruitment was closed early (after enrolling 460 out of a planned 600) for concern for harm per preplanned analysis of deaths within the first 48 hours. These deaths tended to be in the smallest and most vulnerable infants.
- No difference in composite death or BPD at 36 weeks' PMA was detected between the sustained inflation group (63.7%) and the standard resuscitation group (59.2%) (adjusted relative risk 1.1, 95% CI 0.9 to 1.2, $p = 0.29$).
- For secondary outcomes, the only differences found were that infants receiving sustained inflation were more likely to have a heart rate less than 60 beats per minute after the first resuscitation maneuver (23.4% vs 11.4%, $p < 0.01$) and death within 48 hours (7.4% vs 1.4%, $p = 0.002$).

Criticisms and Limitations: Ending a trial early is always problematic. First, the trial may have been underpowered. A post hoc Bayesian analysis did suggest that no benefit from sustained inflation would have been uncovered had trial recruitment continued to the target enrollment. However, it has been shown that truncated trials have a tendency toward more extreme results.[4] Moreover, truncated trials often carry a disproportionate amount of weight on a topic, as they can discourage further study. One must acknowledge that the ability to draw definitive conclusions from this trial is necessarily limited.

While those delivering the intervention received extensive training in the study technique, detailed monitoring in the delivery room was not performed, limiting the ability to detect potential differences in the intervention actually provided.

The issue of consent for trials in neonatal resuscitation medicine is worth noting here. Given the urgent and often unpredictable timing of resuscitation interventions, prospective informed consent can be a considerable challenge and a potential threat to trial generalizability. This trial utilized deferred consent at 6 of 18 study sites, followed by full informed consent for ongoing study participation after resuscitation. This approach was justified by the fact that sustained inflation was standard care at some sites.

Other Relevant Studies and Information:
- SAIL enrolled only infants at the extremes of prematurity (23 to 26 weeks' gestation), which was a more immature population than previous trials.
- Foglia et al.[5] performed a meta-analysis for confirmation of the SAIL results from pooled data of gestational age groups. This described heterogeneity based on gestational age subgroups, with younger gestational ages showing increased risk of death with sustained inflation. However, no gestational age subgroup demonstrated a definitive difference in mortality between sustained inflation and control.
- These results led the European Consensus Guidelines to recommend that the use of sustained inflation be restricted to clinical trials.[6]

Summary and Implications: The SAIL trial showed sustained inflation to be of no benefit, and of potential harm, for resuscitation of preterm infants. At the time SAIL was published, sustained inflation was standard practice in parts of Europe. This large and rigorous trial refuted the wisdom largely from animal studies that sustained inflation was beneficial in the resuscitation of preterm infants. The results of this trial led to practice change away from sustained inflation.

A CONVERSATION WITH THE TRIALIST: HARESH KIRPALANI

How confident can we be about the results of the SAIL trial, given the early closure of enrollment? What would be your hopes for future studies?

The subsequent meta-analysis by Foglia appears to me to confirm the overall findings, finding that "sustained inflation was associated with increased risk of death in the first 2 days after birth (risk difference, 3.1%, 95% CI 0.9%–5.3%)." However, the mechanism remains unclear. As for new trials, it would require a brave-hearted group! If one is to be done, it might consider: replicating the animal studies by using SI in intubated infants. This would seem counterintuitive to clinicians trying to avoid having to intubate due to concerns for BPD.

Deferred consent is rarely practiced in US trials, but its use at foreign study sites for SAIL likely strengthened and improved the generalizability of results. Is this a practice you would hope to see more commonly in US trials in neonatal resuscitation?

While it is controversial, I think its broader application in emergent situations is warranted to increase generalizability to especially vulnerable populations. To do this wisely we should have broad community participation in assessing the trade-offs: limited individual consent for a short period versus more meaningful results over a longer period of time.

References

1. Kirpalani H, Ratcliffe SJ, Keszler M, et al. Effect of sustained inflations vs inter-mittent positive pressure ventilation on bronchopulmonary dysplasia or death among extremely preterm infants: the SAIL randomized clinical trial. *JAMA.* 2019;321(12):1165–75.
2. te Pas AB, Siew M, Wallace MJ, et al. Establishing functional residual capacity at birth: the effect of sustained inflation and positive end-expiratory pressure in a pre-term rabbit model. *Pediatr Res.* 2009;65(5):537–41.
3. Sobotka, K., Hooper, S., Allison, B. et al. An initial sustained inflation improves the respiratory and cardiovascular transition at birth in preterm lambs. *Pediatr Res.* 2011;70:56–60.
4. Guyatt GH, Briel M, Glasziou P, et al. Problems of stopping trials early. *BMJ.* 2012;344:e3863.
5. Foglia EE, Te Pas AB, Kirpalani H, et al. Sustained inflation vs standard resuscitation for preterm infants: a systematic review and meta-analysis. *JAMA Pediatr.* 2020;174(4):e195897.
6. Sweet DG, Carnielli V, Greisen G, et al. European consensus guidelines on the management of respiratory distress syndrome - 2019 update. *Neonatology.* 2019;115(4):432–50.

Cardiovascular

6

Effects of Indomethacin in Premature Infants With Patent Ductus Arteriosus

SOUVIK MITRA

"It appears that the preferable treatment in the small premature infant presenting with hemodynamically significant patent ductus arteriosus is to use indomethacin only after an appropriate course of usual medical therapy (e.g., fluid restriction, diuretics, and perhaps digoxin) fails."

—GERSONY ET AL.[1]

Research Question: Among infants weighing ≤1750 g at birth diagnosed with a hemodynamically significant patent ductus arteriosus [PDA], can PDA closure be safely improved by (A) initial indomethacin versus placebo, or (B) in the event that placebo treatment fails, indomethacin versus surgical PDA ligation?

Why Was This Study Done: This was one of the earliest national collaborative studies in the field, and it remains one of the few collaborative studies on this topic.

Year Study Began: 1979

Year Study Published: 1983

Study Location: United States (13 centers)

Who Was Studied: Infants with birth weight ≤1750 g with a hemodynamically significant PDA. Hemodynamic significance was based on a diagnostic scheme of presence of various combinations of murmurs, other cardiopulmonary abnormalities, and laboratory findings.

Who Was Excluded: Infants with a birth weight ≤500 g, congenital anomalies, chromosomal abnormalities, death in the first 24 hours of life, admission to study facility after 14 days of age, or contraindications to indomethacin.

How Many Patients: 421

Study Overview: This was a 2-stage (trials A & B) parallel-group, partially masked RCT (Figure 6.1).

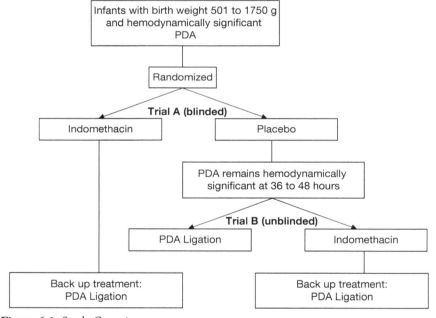

Figure 6.1 Study Overview

What Were the Interventions:
- **Trial A**
  - Infants randomized to the intervention group (one-third of patients) received an intravenous course of indomethacin.
  - Infants randomized to the placebo group received an intravenous course of placebo. All infants were evaluated at 36 to 48 hours, and

if criteria for a significant PDA were still met, infants in the placebo group progressed to **Trial B**:

- Infants randomized at this stage to indomethacin received an intravenous course of indomethacin.
- Infants randomized to ligation underwent surgical PDA ligation.

All randomized infants had a backup treatment option of surgical PDA ligation.

How Long Was Follow-up: Hospital discharge

What Were the Endpoints:
Primary outcome: Primary PDA closure.
Selected secondary outcomes: Death, common complications of prematurity (including BPD, pneumothorax, IVH, NEC, advanced ROP).

Concerns Regarding Bias: This trial was at high risk for performance/detection bias in Trial B, as caregivers were not blinded to the intervention.

RESULTS

- Infants who received usual medical therapy and indomethacin had a significantly higher primary PDA closure rate compared with usual medical therapy alone (79% versus 35%; p <0.001).
- When indomethacin was used as a backup therapy for infants who failed to respond to medical therapy alone (trial B), 27% ultimately underwent PDA ligation (as compared with 21% of infants originally treated with indomethacin).
- Of several secondary outcomes, pneumothorax (39% versus 15%; p <0.001) and ROP (15% versus 4%; $p = 0.02$) were significantly higher in the surgical PDA ligation group compared with the initial indomethacin group. No statistically significant differences were noted for mortality, BPD, IVH, or NEC between any of the 3 groups.

Criticisms and Limitations: In this study, the improvement in PDA closure with indomethacin failed to translate into clinically meaningful benefits such as reduction in mortality, BPD, IVH, or NEC. However, we cannot definitively conclude from this study that PDA closure does not improve clinical outcomes. First, all randomized infants had the backup option of surgical PDA closure regardless of their allocation, if the PDA remained open.

Second, no sample size was prespecified in this trial, making interpretation of secondary outcomes difficult.

Third, the diagnosis of hemodynamically significant PDA was based primarily on clinical criteria, and echocardiographic confirmation of hemodynamic significance was not mandatory. After this trial was published, clinical signs of PDA were shown to be unreliable and inaccurate.[2,3] Therefore, generalizability of trial results to current-day practices is unclear—but is largely supported by the results of the Cochrane review.[4]

Other Relevant Studies and Information:
- Fourteen small inadequately powered RCTs comparing indomethacin with placebo or no treatment have been conducted to date. However pooling results in a Cochrane systematic review and meta-analysis largely align with the results of this single trial.[4] From the meta-analysis, there was high-certainty evidence to conclude that indomethacin was effective in closing a symptomatic PDA compared with placebo or no treatment. However, there was no evidence supporting the effects of indomethacin on other clinically relevant outcomes and medication-related adverse effects.
- A recent multicenter RCT of another cyclo-oxygenase inhibitor used for PDA closure (ibuprofen) does not support the need for early treatment. The authors found expectant management to be noninferior to early ibuprofen for the composite outcome of NEC, BPD, or death at 36 weeks' PMA.[5]

Summary and Implications: This national collaborative RCT showed that indomethacin in preterm infants with clinical signs of a hemodynamically significant PDA was superior in closing the PDA to usual therapy. However, when considering indomethacin therapy in preterm infants, the benefits of PDA closure should be weighed against the lack of demonstrated efficacy in altering clinical outcomes.

A CONVERSATION WITH THE TRIALIST: WELTON M. GERSONY

Do you think the clinical outcomes would have been different had backup surgery not been allowed in the control group?

Yes. Even in retrospect after 40 years, the criteria for surgical intervention in the National Collaborative study appear to be reasonable. Perhaps today, they could be more stringent. However, if a premature infant is in heart failure with a massive left to right shunt due to a large patent ductus, it would be hard to argue that closing the ductus would not be indicated, nor that survival would not be much more likely.

Do you think further trials will be able to clarify this apparent disconnect between PDA closure and downstream clinical benefits, through better patient selection or other means?

It is quite remarkable that after 4 decades, many issues regarding ductal closure remain unresolved. Of course, more data is always useful. However, it seems to be clear that conservative "watchful waiting" without aggressive medical or surgical intervention is the reasonable approach. Large PDAs with heart failure should be closed. Further trials would have to be massive and complex, and are not likely to be worth the commitment of expensive resources.

References

1. Gersony WM, Peckham GJ, Ellison RC, et al. Effects of indomethacin in premature infants with patent ductus arteriosus: results of a national collaborative study. *J Pediatr.* 1983 Jun;102(6):895–906.
2. Davis P, Turner-Gomes S, Cunningham K, et al. Precision and accuracy of clinical and radiological signs in premature infants at risk of patent ductus arteriosus. *Arch Pediatr Adolesc Med.* 1995 Oct;149(10):1136–41.
3. Skelton R, Evans N, Smythe J. A blinded comparison of clinical and echocardiographic evaluation of the preterm infant for patent ductus arteriosus. *J Paediatr Child Health.* 1994 Oct;30(5):406–11.
4. Evans P, O'Reilly D, Flyer JN, et al. Indomethacin for symptomatic patent ductus arteriosus in preterm infants. *Cochrane Database Syst Rev.* 2021 Jan 15;1:CD013133.
5. Hundscheid T, Onland W, Kooi EMW, et al; BeNeDuctus Trial Investigators. Expectant management or early ibuprofen for patent ductus arteriosus. *NEJM.* 2023;388(11):980–90.

Extracorporeal Circulation in Neonatal Respiratory Failure

ELIZABETH BAKER AND PETER G. DAVIS

"The 'randomized play-the-winner' method was appropriate for this study because the outcome of each case is usually known within a few days after the assigned treatment begins, so that the odds of subsequent random assignment can be adjusted. This method softened the ethical dilemma, although withholding ECMO from the control patient still caused controversy."

—BARTLETT ET AL.[1]

Research Question: Does extracorporeal membrane oxygenation (ECMO) compared with conventional therapy decrease mortality in newborns with a birth weight >2 kg and respiratory failure in the first week after birth?

Why Was This Study Done: At the time of this trial, ECMO had been successfully used in several centers to treat respiratory failure. While safety and efficacy were still being evaluated by Phase I trials, there was already loss of equipoise in favor of ECMO,[2,3] with an anticipated dramatically improved survival.

Year Study Began: 1982

Year Study Published: 1985

Study Location: United States (1 center)

Who Was Studied: Infants with birth weight >2 kg and severe respiratory failure in the first week after birth, who were not responsive to "optimal standard therapy" and at ≥80% risk of mortality.[4]

Who Was Excluded: Infants with grade ≥II intracranial hemorrhage, older than 7 days, or those anticipated to have severe neurological impairment (e.g., those experiencing prolonged cardiac arrest).

How Many Patients: 12

Study Overview: This parallel-group, unmasked RCT was based on a "play-the-winner" statistical method.[5] In this method, the likelihood of randomization to a particular treatment arm depended on the prior success of that arm. For example, the more that infants survived after receiving ECMO, the more likely it became that the next infant would be randomized to ECMO (Figure 7.1).

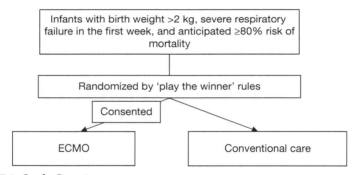

Figure 7.1 Study Overview

What Were the Interventions:
- Infants randomized to the ECMO group received either venovenous or venoarterial (if hemodynamically unstable) bypass and ECMO performed with a Sci-Med membrane lung. Once stable on ECMO, ventilator settings were decreased to allow for "lung rest;" then as lung function improved, flow through the extracorporeal system was weaned. Infants were decannulated when normal gas exchange was maintained on low ventilator and ECMO settings.
- Infants randomized to the control group continued with conventional care; including muscle relaxation, pulmonary vasodilation, and inotropic support as indicated.

How Long Was Follow-up: Hospital discharge

What Were the Endpoints:
Primary outcome: Death.
Selected secondary outcomes: Time on ECMO, complications including intracranial hemorrhage, time to extubation, length of hospital stay.

Concerns Regarding Bias: This unique design can introduce possible selection bias, as only those randomized to the intervention were consented. Additionally, though statisticians generating the randomization sequence were blinded, other researchers were not blinded to outcomes and were likely increasingly aware that the likelihood of allocation to the ECMO arm increased as the trial progressed. This knowledge may have influenced the decision to enroll selected infants. There was also high risk for performance/observer bias, as blinding could not be performed.

RESULTS

- Only 12 infants were studied. All 11 infants who received ECMO survived. The single infant who received standard therapy died.
- ECMO-related complications occurred in 3 patients; these were intracerebral hemorrhage, rupture of the jugular vein during cannulation, and fault in ECMO equipment.
- At least 4 infants had adverse neurological sequelae, the nature of which is unclear.

Criticisms and Limitations: The authors designed a randomized study that attempted to deal with the ethical conundrum of withholding potentially life-saving treatment. To do this, they employed the novel "play-the-winner" randomization strategy. This study was highly criticized at the time (". . . the results are not completely convincing. Why not? Primarily because only one patient received standard therapy . . ."[6]) and labelled by some as a failure.[7]

The novel study design is difficult to interpret. Although meeting the criteria for success, the risk of selection, performance, and observer biases are important and compromise the study. Furthermore, the predefined "stopping rule" resulted in a very small number of infants enrolled, limiting the precision of the study. Beyond the biases, the limited numbers do not allow for any analysis of safety. If a new therapy is to be widely adopted, the recruitment of one infant to the control arm is likely unconvincing.

Other Relevant Studies and Information:

- Two subsequent small trials (one using conventional randomization, the other using an adaptive approach) supported these initial findings.[8,9]
- The global neonatal community proceeded in different directions subsequent to this published evidence on ECMO.[10] Whereas ECMO centers proliferated in the United States, the United Kingdom formed a large trial group to definitively assess ECMO by conventional RCT (the UK ECMO trial, detailed in Chapter 8).
- A systematic review that included this small trial and the large UK trial, along with 2 other trials, ultimately supported the impressive impact of ECMO on mortality in infants with severe respiratory failure (RR 0.44, 95% CI 0.31 to 0.61).[11]
- The trial authors established the Extracorporeal Life Support Organization (ELSO), a registry that now includes almost 200,000 cases (including almost 50,000 newborns) allowing follow-up for safety and longer-term complications.[12]

Summary and Implications: This trial generated much controversy. In performing an adaptive trial, the authors attempted to balance providing a perceived "randomized" design with a strongly perceived ethical dilemma of not withholding innovative but unproven "heroic" and expensive therapy. However, given the deficiencies discussed above, this trial was perceived by many as a "failure" and is said to be responsible for adaptive trial designs falling out of favor at the time.[8] Despite its controversies, the conclusion drawn by Bartlett and colleagues, that ECMO decreases mortality in term infants with severe respiratory failure, has been supported by subsequent studies.

A CONVERSATION WITH THE TRIALIST: ROBERT H. BARTLETT

We had the unique opportunity for a longer conversation with trialist, Robert H. Bartlett. His story is fascinating, as a driving force behind ECMO as used in neonatology today. He described using ECMO for adults as a general surgeon, with development of the technique for application to neonates and publishing a series of case reports demonstrating dramatic improvement in survival. Facets of ECMO protocol that continue to this day, including the Oxygenation Index, used to determine ECMO candidacy, were invented by his team. Acknowledging both the need for proof beyond case reports and the ethical conundrum of denying this likely life-saving treatment to a group of infants in a classical RCT, he approached statistician Richard Cornell, and the two strategized a way to apply the Play-the-Winner technique in the form of a blinded prospective RCT. Per Bartlett, "At the time it was considered crazy and outrageous, and now it's considered pretty standard."

Bartlett described the team's ethical struggle of not putting the one infant randomized to conventional treatment on ECMO ("The trial should be more important than this baby who is probably going to die, and that's worse when you're the investigator."), with both relief and misgivings at the rapid termination of the trial for statistical significance: "I said, 'No one is going to believe this.' . . . It was published in *Pediatrics*, along with flaming letters." He went on to collaborate with one of his strongest critics, who ultimately published the second adaptive trial on ECMO.

Bartlett was key in establishing the ELSO registry, providing further evidence for the safety and efficacy ECMO use for neonates: "Starting in the 80s, we taught people how to do ECMO. . . . We didn't charge them, but we said if you do this clinically, please let us know what happened." He set the standard of what it meant to bring a community together, as both a trialist and a visionary.

References

1. Bartlett RH, Roloff D, Cornell RG, et al. Extracorporal circulation in neonatal respiratory failure: a prospective randomized study. *Pediatrics*. 1985;76(4):479–87.
2. Bartlett RH, Gazzaniga AB, Jefferies MR, et al. Extracorporeal membrane oxygenation (ECMO) cardiopulmonary support in infancy. *Transactions - American Society for Artificial Internal Organs*. 1976;22:80–93.
3. Bartlett RH, Andrews AF, Toomasian JM, et al. Extracorporeal membrane oxygenation for newborn respiratory failure: forty-five cases. *Surgery*. 1982;92(2):425–33.
4. Bartlett RH, Gazzaniga AB, Huxtable RF, et al. Extracorporeal circulation (ECMO) in neonatal respiratory failure. *Cardiovasc Surg*. 1977 Dec;74(6):826–33.
5. Wei LJ, Durham S. The randomized play-the-winner rule in medical trials. *J Am Statist Assoc*. 1978;73(364):840–3.
6. Ware JH, Epstein MF. Extracorporeal circulation in neonatal respiratory failure: a prospective randomized study. *Pediatrics*. 1985;76(5):849–50.
7. Rosenberger WF. Randomized play-the-winner clinical trials: review and recommendations. *Control Clinl Trials*. 1999;20:328–43.
8. O'Rourke PP, Crone RK, Vacanti JP, et al. Extracorporeal membrane oxygenation and conventional medical therapy in neonates with persistent pulmonary hypertension of the newborn: a prospective randomized study. *Pediatrics*. 1989;84(6):957–63.
9. Bifano EM, Hakanson DO, Hingre RV, et al. Prospective randomized controlled trial of conventional treatment or transport for ECMO in infants with persistent pulmonary hypertension (PPHN). *Pediatr Res*. 1992;31:196A.

10. Soll RF. Neonatal extracorporeal membrane oxygenation--a bridging technique. Lancet. 1996 Jul 13;348(9020):70–1.

11. Mugford M, Elbourne D, Field D. Extracorporeal membrane oxygenation for severe respiratory failure in newborn infants. *Cochrane Database Syst Rev.* 2008(3):CD001340.

12. Extracorporeal Life Support Organization. (2023). Registry of Active ELSO Centers Using ECMO. https://www.elso.org/registry.aspx.

8

UK Collaborative Randomized Trial of Neonatal Extracorporeal Membrane Oxygenation

The UK Collaborative ECMO Trial

BRIANNA LIBERIO AND CLYDE J. WRIGHT

"These preliminary results demonstrate the clinical effectiveness of a well-staffed and organized neonatal ECMO service. ECMO support should be actively considered for neonates with severe but potentially reversible respiratory failure."
—UK COLLABORATIVE ECMO TRIAL GROUP[1]

Research Question: Among late preterm and term infants with severe respiratory failure, does a policy of referral to specialist centers for consideration of extracorporeal membrane oxygenation (ECMO), in comparison to conventional management without transfer, improve survival to one year without severe disability?

Why Was This Study Done: Prior to this trial, evidence to support ECMO in newborns with severe respiratory failure was limited to small studies. Approaches to adoption of this technique varied widely across the global community, balancing concerns about cost-effectiveness and long-term disability in survivors.

Year Study Began: 1993

Year Study Published: 1996

Study Location: United Kingdom (55 centers; ECMO performed at 5 centers)

Who Was Studied: Late preterm or term infants (gestational age ≥35 weeks) within the first 28 days of life and with birth weight ≥2 kg, who had severe respiratory failure (defined by oxygenation index ≥40, arterial partial pressure of carbon dioxide >12 kPa [90 mm Hg] for at least 3 hours) and received high-pressure ventilation for <10 days.

Who Was Excluded: Infants with a contraindication for ECMO support (e.g., ventricular hemorrhage, irreversible cardiopulmonary disease); or potential grounds for treatment withdrawal (i.e., major congenital or chromosomal anomaly, severe encephalopathy).

How Many Patients: 185. Of note, the study target sample size was 300. Recruitment was terminated early (November 1995) after planned interim analysis demonstrated a clear advantage with ECMO.

Study Overview: The UK Collaborative ECMO Trial was a parallel-group, unmasked RCT (Figure 8.1).

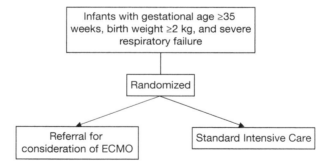

Figure 8.1 Study Overview

What Were the Interventions:
- Patients randomized to the intervention group were transported to an ECMO center. If the patient's condition was judged to be appropriate for ECMO, the patient was cannulated and ECMO was initiated as soon as possible. Venoarterial (VA) and venovenous (VV) ECMO were both permitted. Once weaned off ECMO, decannulated, and stable, most patients were transferred back to the original referring hospital.

- Patients randomized to the conventional management group received standard intensive care at the referring hospital.

How Long Was Follow-up: 1 year

What Were the Endpoints:
Primary outcome: Composite outcome of death or severe disability (defined as an overall developmental quotient of <50 using the Griffiths Mental Development Scales (GMDS), or blindness, or level of function prohibiting GMDS evaluation) at 1 year of age.
Selected secondary outcomes: Economic evaluation, including a cost-effectiveness analysis.

Concerns Regarding Bias: The trial was at high risk for performance/detection bias, as caregivers were not blinded to the intervention. However, blinding of the developmental pediatrician at time of neurodevelopmental assessment was achieved. There is additionally an unclear risk of bias because of the early termination. Moreover, possible other cointerventions from transfer to a high intensity NICU may have occurred.

RESULTS

- For the primary outcome, patients in the ECMO group had a lower rate of the composite outcome of death or severe disability at 1 year of age (33% versus 62%; relative risk [RR] 0.54, 95% confidence interval [CI] 0.36 to 0.80, $p = 0.002$). At the time of publication, the data for the composite outcome of death or severe disability (primary outcome) was known only for those enrolled by Dec. 1, 1994 ($n = 124$).
- Patients in the ECMO group had a lower rate of mortality up to 1 year of age (32% versus 59%; RR 0.55, 95% CI 0.39 to 0.77, $p = 0.0005$). This equates to 1 extra survivor for every 3 to 4 patients allocated to ECMO.

Criticisms and Limitations: The authors acknowledged that the differences in outcomes could be overestimates because ECMO providers could have been more enthusiastic about this newer technology or could have had greater experience providing such intensive care, as compared with the conventional management providers. Additionally, possible cointerventions may have occurred as those randomized to the standard intensive care group did not receive care at the ECMO center. One commentary criticized the trial design for allowing subjects randomized to standard care to remain at the referring hospital.[2] It was argued that this design introduced variability in management that would have been avoided by sending all recruited patients to the ECMO centers, regardless of whether they were to receive standard care or ECMO. In the original manuscript, the authors justified this saying referral hospitals had to meet certain experience criteria, and there was no difference found between teaching and nonteaching referral hospitals. Finally, the authors proposed that the advantages of ECMO could have been underestimated due to the inherent risks of transporting a critically ill newborn and the delay to ECMO initiation.

The timing of this trial in the history of ECMO has drawn criticism, as the technique was already widely in use in the United States at this time, supported by adaptive trial evidence (See play-the-winner ECMO trial, detailed in Chapter 7) and registry data without suggestion of catastrophic outcomes. Arguably, this trial's place in history could have been closer to the introduction of ECMO for use in infants in 1976, not 2 decades later.[3]

Other Relevant Studies and Information:
- A subsequent manuscript reported the primary outcome of death or severe disability at 1 year for the full sample of 185 patients, with results continuing to favor the ECMO group.[4]
- Economic evaluation was reported in a later manuscript.[5] While the policy of referral for ECMO consideration increased the cost of neonatal health care, it was concluded that this was likely to be as cost-effective as other life-extending technologies.
- The cohort of survivors was followed at 4 years of age and 7 years of age, with results showing that the policy of referral for ECMO consideration remained effective in reducing death or severe disability as compared with conventional management for infants with severe respiratory failure.[6,7]
- A 2008 Cochrane Systematic Review included 4 RCTs comparing ECMO to conventional management in neonates with severe respiratory failure. All 4 trials showed a significant benefit of ECMO on mortality.[8]
- From the Extracorporeal Life Support Organization registry, neonatal ECMO cases had peaked at >1500 cases around the start of the present trial. Neonatal ECMO cases have gradually declined in number. Authors of the present trial propose improvements in obstetric and neonatal intensive care as contributors to this decline; including increased use of surfactant, inhaled nitric oxide, and less aggressive ventilator strategies.[9]

Summary and Implications: For infants with severe respiratory failure, the UK Collaborative ECMO Trial showed a significant advantage on survival without severe disability following a policy of referral for ECMO consideration compared with conventional management. At a time when the concern for long-term effects of ECMO in neonates was causing hesitation in its use, the results from this study, as well as consistent follow-up results at 4 and 7 years of age, encouraged the development of neonatal ECMO services around the world. This study also demonstrated that large, rigorous RCTs of emergency life-saving treatment are feasible.

A CONVERSATION WITH THE TRIALIST: DAVID FIELD

Could you discuss the ethical questions that arose in designing this trial? Do you think that other stakeholders would have different views of how much evidence is required before adoption?

The ethical issues clearly loomed large! There were staunch believers in ECMO and there were those who effectively felt it should not be used, as if it worked to save life it simply produced damaged babies—plenty in both camps. The Government would not fund it without strong evidence. You get a sense of all this if you look at some of the letters to the BMJ (might have been the Lancet too as well as some newspaper articles) in the run-up to the Trial. In the end there was a pretty broad consensus that the way to deal with these issues was a trial.

References

1. UK Collaborative ECMO Trial Group. UK collaborative randomised trial of neonatal extracorporeal membrane oxygenation. *Lancet.* 1996;348:75–82.
2. Shann F. UK trial of extracorporeal membrane oxygenation gave biased estimate of efficacy. *BMJ.* 1999 Mar 13;318(7185):738.
3. Soll RF. Neonatal extracorporeal membrane oxygenation--a bridging technique. *Lancet.* 1996 Jul 13;348(9020):70–1.
4. UK Collaborative ECMO Trial Group. The Collaborative UK ECMO Trial: follow-up at 1 year of age. *Pediatrics.* 1998 April;101(4):E1.
5. Roberts TE; Extracorporeal Membrane Oxygenation Economics Working Group. Economic evaluation and randomised controlled trial of extracorporeal membrane oxygenation: UK collaborative trial. *BMJ.* 1998 Oct 3;317(7163):911–16.
6. Bennett CC, Johnson A, Field DJ, et al.; UK Collaborative ECMO Trial Group. UK collaborative randomised trial of neonatal extracorporeal membrane oxygenation: follow-up to age 4 years. *Lancet.* 2001 Apr 7;357(9262):1094–6.

7. McNally H, Bennett CC, Elbourne D, et al.; UK Collaborative ECMO Trial Group. UK collaborative randomized trial of neonatal extracorporeal membrane oxygenation: follow-up to age 7 years. *Pediatrics*. 2006 May;117(5):e845–54.

8. Mugford M, Elbourne D, Field D. Extracorporeal membrane oxygenation for severe respiratory failure in newborn infants. *Cochrane Database Syst Rev*. 2008;(3): CD001340.

9. Macrae DJ, Field DJ. Our study 20 years on: UK collaborative randomised trial of neonatal extracorporeal membrane oxygenation. *Intensive Care Med*. 2016 May;42(5):841–43.

9

Inhaled Nitric Oxide in Full-Term and Nearly Full-Term Infants With Hypoxic Respiratory Failure

The NINOS Trial

DIRK BASSLER

"Inhaled nitric oxide reduced the use of extracorporeal membrane oxygenation in critically ill neonates born at or near term with hypoxic respiratory failure who had received maximal conventional therapy."
—THE NINOS GROUP[1]

Research Question: Among full-term and nearly full-term infants with severe hypoxic respiratory failure, does a strategy including inhaled nitric oxide (iNO), compared with 100%, oxygen, reduce the incidence of extracorporeal membrane oxygenation (ECMO) or mortality by 120 days?

Why Was This Study Done: Nitric oxide regulates vascular tone and was hypothesized to reverse persistent pulmonary hypertension, a condition at the time with no effective therapies known to reduce need for ECMO or mortality. Prior to this trial, iNO was evaluated in several small studies with inconsistent results.

Year Study Began: Not stated

Year Study Published: 1997

Study Location: United States (12 centers), Canada (9 centers)

Who Was Studied: Infants born at ≥34 weeks' gestation who required assisted ventilation for hypoxic respiratory failure, with an oxygenation index (OI) ≥25.

Who Was Excluded: Infants >14 days, with congenital diaphragmatic hernia, known congenital heart disease, or with a decision not to provide full treatment.

How Many Patients: 235. The study was powered on a sample of 250, but was terminated early for efficacy at the recommendation of the Data Safety and Monitoring Committee after the second planned interim analysis.

Study Overview: The NINOS trial was a parallel-group, masked RCT (Figure 9.1).

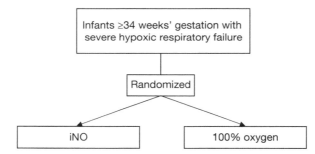

Figure 9.1 Study Overview

What Were the Interventions:
- Infants randomized to iNO received therapy-grade nitric oxide. iNO was started at 20 ppm, with option to increase to a maximal dose of 80 ppm in the setting of incomplete response (defined as <20 mm Hg increase in the partial pressure of oxygen in the arterial blood [PaO_2]).
- Infants randomized to oxygen received 100% oxygen.

Study drug titration was guided by suggested algorithms, which allowed courses up to 14 days.

The general approach to care was not standardized between centers, including criteria for ECMO. Each center developed its own management guideline, with agreement to use the most aggressive forms of conventional therapy prior to randomization. No crossover was allowed between the 2 treatment groups.

How Long Was Follow-up: 120 days

What Were the Endpoints:
Primary outcome: Composite outcome of death by 120 days or the initiation of ECMO.
Selected secondary outcomes: Components of the primary outcome, duration of assisted ventilation, incidence of air leakage, safety outcomes (including blood methemoglobin concentrations).

Concerns Regarding Bias: Despite this being a trial testing a drug-delivery device bedside, efforts appeared successful in blinding caregivers to intervention. The early termination of study enrollment may be a source of bias.[2] While the drug was provided by industry, all scientific decisions, including the design of the trial, were made independently.

RESULTS

- iNO reduced the incidence of death or ECMO (46% versus 64%; $p = 0.006$).
- This reduction was mainly due to a decrease in ECMO (39% versus 55%; $p = 0.014$), with no statistically significant difference between groups in mortality (16% versus 20%; $p = 0.60$). The causes of death in the 2 groups did not differ.
- There was no difference in the duration of assisted ventilation or incidence of air leak.
- There was no discontinuation of the study drug for toxic effects.

Criticisms and Limitations: NINOS was designed as a management trial, presenting an algorithm to dictate titrations of iNO for hypoxic respiratory failure. This careful design provided a basis for subsequent practice recommendations around iNO, but the outcome measures studied left the response to iNO less clear.

As in prior studies of iNO in late-preterm and term infants, infants met strict criteria for neonatal hypoxic respiratory failure and therefore were at high risk of mortality. However, no decrease in death is reported, with the possibility of ECMO potentially circumventing death as a meaningful primary outcome. The benefits of iNO were in reducing the use of ECMO. However, in this trial, this was a subjective outcome, as thresholds for ECMO initiation were left to the discretion of participating centers. Additionally, the question of what iNO may accomplish in healthcare settings without easy access to ECMO remains unanswered.

Of note, as in other trials, there is always concern for overestimating efficacy when a study is stopped early.

Other Relevant Studies and Information:
- iNO is the only FDA-approved pulmonary vasodilator widely accepted as a standard of care in the management of hypoxic respiratory failure in developed countries. This treatment in full-term and nearly full-term infants is not associated with an increase in neurodevelopmental, behavioral, or medical abnormalities at 2 years of age.[3]
- Despite treatment drift with an increasing use in younger populations (with almost half of its use occurring in preterm infants by 2010),[4] the evidence of benefits of iNO as an effective rescue therapy for preterm babies (≤34 weeks' gestation) with severe hypoxic respiratory failure is more controversial.[5]

Summary and Implications: The NINOS trial showed that iNO reduced the use of ECMO, but had no apparent effect on mortality, in critically ill full-term and nearly full-term infants with hypoxic respiratory failure. The study was designed as a management trial and serves as the basis of current practice recommendations.

A CONVERSATION WITH THE TRIALIST: NEIL FINER

The NINOS trial was successful in treating late-preterm and term infants with hypoxic respiratory failure. What are your thoughts on the use of iNO in other populations, including the preterm population or the term population with congenital diaphragmatic hernia (CDH)?

It is important to note that none of the larger RCTs evaluating iNO in the hypoxic preterm infant required a pretreatment echocardiogram assessment. That said, an individualized approach to such infants is discussed by the NIH Consensus Development Conference statement on iNO and preterm infants, as well as the guidelines provided by the American Thoracic Society and the Pediatric Pulmonary Hypertension group.[1-3]

... For the preterm infant, if the infant has unresponsive hypoxia and the care team is considering the use of iNO, I would recommend an immediate and thorough echocardiogram by an experienced individual to rule out congenital heart disease before starting, and if the decision is made to use iNO, start with a very small dose ....

As for CDH, the RCTs have not demonstrated that iNO is associated with a reduction in mortality or need for ECMO, I would again emphasize the need for a full diagnostic echocardiogram and repeated assessments depending on the clinical situation—it is critically important to evaluate left ventricular function in such infants. Infants with CDH can have recurrent severe pulmonary hypertension postoperatively, and in this setting iNO may improve oxygenation.[4] I am unclear if further RCTs in these populations will prove informative as the variation in infants and their management is significant.

1. Cole FS, Alleyne C, Barks JDE, et al. NIH Consensus Development Conference statement: inhaled nitric-oxide therapy for premature infants. *Pediatrics* 2011;127(2):363–69.
2. Abman SH, Hansmann Georg, Archer SL, et al. Pediatric pulmonary hypertension: guidelines from the American Heart Association and American Thoracic Society. *Circulation* 2015;132(21):2037–99
3. Kinsella JP, Steinhorn RH, Krishnan US, et al. Recommendations for the use of inhaled nitric oxide therapy in premature newborns with severe pulmonary hypertension. *J Pediatr* 2016;170:312–14.
4. Kinsella JP, Ivy DD, Abman SH. Pulmonary vasodilator therapy in congenital diaphragmatic hernia: acute, late, and chronic pulmonary hypertension. *Semin Perinatology* 2005;29(2):123–8.

References

1. Neonatal Inhaled Nitric Oxide Study Group. Inhaled nitric oxide in full-term and nearly full-term infants with hypoxic respiratory failure. *N Engl J Med.* 1997;336(9):597–604.
2. Bassler D, Briel M, Montori VM, et al. Stopping randomized trials early for benefit and estimation of treatment effects: systematic review and meta-regression analysis. *JAMA.* 2010 Mar 24;303(12):1180–7.
3. Neonatal Inhaled Nitric Oxide Study Group. Inhaled nitric oxide in term and near-term infants: neurodevelopmental follow-up of the neonatal inhaled nitric oxide study group (NINOS). *J Pediatr.* 2000 May;136(5):611–7.
4. Ellsworth MA, Harris MN, Carey WA, et al. Off-label use of inhaled nitric oxide after release of NIH consensus statement. *Pediatrics.* 2015 Apr;135(4):643–8.
5. Barrington KJ, Finer N, Pennaforte T. Inhaled nitric oxide for respiratory failure in preterm infants. *Cochrane Database Syst Rev.* 2017 Jan 3;1(1):CD000509.

Respiratory

10

Prevention of Neonatal Respiratory Distress Syndrome by Tracheal Instillation of Surfactant

COLM P.F. O'DONNELL

" . . . surfactant supplementation prior to the first breath is feasible and is of value as protection against the respiratory distress syndrome and the negative effects of hypoxia and ventilator support."

—ENHORNING ET AL.[1]

Research Question: Among infants born <30 weeks' gestation who are intubated at birth, does instilling a surfactant suspension extracted from calf lungs, as compared with a sham injection of air, improve oxygenation in the first 72 hours of life?

Why Was This Study Done: Surfactant deficiency was the suspected etiology of respiratory distress syndrome (RDS) since 1959.[2] However, it took decades of bench and animal work to approach a safe and effective means of replacing this surfactant, with a 10-infant study demonstrating the feasibility of endotracheal instillation of surfactant 5 years prior to this publication.[3]

Year Study Began: Not stated

Year Study Published: 1985

Study Location: Canada (single center)

Who Was Studied: Infants born <30 weeks' gestation who were intubated at birth

Who Was Excluded: Exclusion criteria were not specified; 2 infants with congenital anomalies (esophageal atresia and myotubular myopathy) and 2 infants with "possible pulmonary hypoplasia" were included. Consent for participation was sought before birth; mothers were not approached for consent "if they were in danger of imminent delivery or were under the influence of hypnotic medication."

How Many Patients: 72

Study Overview: This study was a parallel-group, masked RCT, with randomization stratified by gestational age (<27 weeks, 27 to 29 weeks) and receipt of antenatal steroids (complete, partial, none) (Figure 10.1).

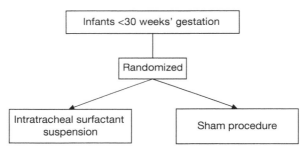

Figure 10.1 Study Overview

What Were the Interventions:
- Infants randomized to surfactant received a surfactant suspension extracted by the investigators from calf lungs. This was given directly into the trachea via an endotracheal tube shortly after birth, ideally "before the first breath."
- Infants randomized to the sham procedure received an intratracheal injection of air.

How Long Was Follow-up: Hospital discharge

What Were the Endpoints:
Primary outcomes: The arterial/alveolar (a/A) PO$_2$ ratio; measured by arterial blood gas sampling during the first 72 hours of life.

Selected secondary outcomes: Other oxygenation parameters (difference between alveolar and arterial PO$_2$ [A-a DO$_2$], oxygen hours, ventilation index [peak inspiratory pressure × frequency]), RDS, pulmonary interstitial emphysema (PIE), mortality.

Concerns Regarding Bias: The study was at unclear risk for performance/ascertainment bias. Although a sham procedure was used and "attempts were thus made to 'blind' the study, . . . these attempts may not always have been completely successful."

RESULTS

- The a/A ratio was on average 0.15 higher in the surfactant group over the first 72 hours of life ($p < 0.05$).
- Other oxygenation parameters (A-a DO$_2$, oxygen hours, ventilation index) also demonstrated improvement with surfactant over the first 72 hours.
- Fewer treated infants had PIE on chest radiographs (3 versus 13; $p < 0.005$).
- Fewer treated infants died in the neonatal period (1 versus 6; $p < 0.05$); although there was no significant difference in total death, with one additional death beyond the neonatal period reported in each group.

Criticisms and Limitations: This RCT was ambitious in its time as it involved a delivery room intervention of an innovative product. It paid attention to stratification and the importance of antenatal corticosteroid treatment in enrolled mothers. The number of participants is small, although appropriately so, as the trial was designed to test the efficacy of this new therapy as hypothesized in the lab. As in all surfactant trials, blinding poses a unique challenge and potential entry point for bias.

This was one of the first trials to show immediate effects of surfactant on lung damage (which would be proven later in meta-analysis; see Other Relevant Studies and Information). However, the authors noted no improvement in BPD, and they questioned whether the definition used (requirement of supplemental oxygen beyond 30 days) was adequate. This group would later develop the definition of BPD as requirement of supplemental oxygen at 36 weeks' PMA,[4] the subsequent standard.

Other Relevant Studies and Information:
- The authors published long-term follow-up of the participants, and found a reduced rate of death but not of neurodevelopmental handicap at 2 years.[5]
- Initial meta-analyses showed a decrease in pneumothoraces and a combined decrease in BPD or death.[6]
- Surfactant was incorporated into standard of care by the 1990s, revolutionizing treatment and the subsequent outcomes for infants born prematurely.[7]
- This study employed aggressive pre-ventilatory surfactant administration, in keeping with earlier animal evidence demonstrating superior lung distribution with this method.[8] However, subsequent studies demonstrated that this pre-ventilatory timing may not be necessary.[9]
- With continued advances of NICU care, the relative benefit of surfactant was revisited, with results supportive of selective use (See SUPPORT, Chapter 15). The role of surfactant and alternative means of delivery continue to evolve.

Summary and Implications: This ground-breaking study demonstrated that it was feasible to perform a RCT that enrolled infants at birth, that it was possible to give surfactant prepared from calf lungs to preterm infants who were intubated immediately after birth, and that giving surfactant resulted in improved oxygenation in the first 72 hours of life. The authors also demonstrated an associated reduction in the PIE and deaths in the neonatal period. This added to the growing body of evidence supporting surfactant replacement therapy for the prevention and treatment of preterm infants with RDS.

A CONVERSATION WITH THE TRIALIST: MICHAEL DUNN (CO-AUTHOR OF THIS TRIAL, LEAD AUTHOR OF THE 2-YEAR FOLLOW-UP INVESTIGATION)

Your group went on to refine the definition of BPD; did this particular trial influence that further work?

When examining the outcomes of the babies in this trial, it was evident that the traditional way of defining BPD (i.e., requirement for supplemental O_2 beyond 28 or 30 days) was inappropriate for the population we were studying. With babies born at less than 30 weeks' gestation and especially those born before 27 weeks', it was clear that many would require supplemental oxygen beyond 30 days but we felt this was more related to immaturity and often not a marker of significant lung injury. In *the discussion of this paper, we propose using requirement for supplemental oxygen at 36 weeks' CGA as a better indicator of true BPD.*

Your later work has challenged the aggressive use of prophylactic surfactant. Is there still a patient population for whom you would take this approach?

Dr. Enhorning strongly believed that exogenous surfactant would be most effective if given before the first breath and thus deposited at the air–liquid interface prior to lung aeration. This is the main reason that he approached us to do this trial as we routinely intubated and ventilated all babies born at less than 30 weeks during this epoch. With the results of our trial and a group of studies looking at prophylactic versus rescue surfactant treatment, many clinicians adopted the practice of surfactant prophylaxis for small preterm babies. However, subsequent investigations (including the Vermont Oxford Network Delivery Room Management Trial) revealed that, if CPAP was provided as a primary mode of respiratory support with surfactant given selectively to only those babies showing signs of significant RDS, intubation and prophylactic surfactant was unnecessary and actually inferior. These studies included very preterm babies born [at] less than 30 weeks' gestation, and the SUPPORT trial included those born as early as 24–25 weeks' for whom the advantages of a "CPAP first" approach were also demonstrated. Yet there is little evidence to support trying CPAP first in babies born at less than 24 weeks' in whom the requirement of invasive ventilation is almost universal even if CPAP is effective for a period of time.

References

1. Enhorning G, Shennan A, Possmayer F, et al. Prevention of neonatal respiratory distress syndrome by tracheal instillation of surfactant: a randomized clinical trial. *Pediatrics.* 1985 Aug;76(2):145–53.
2. Avery ME, Mead J. Surface properties in relation to atelectasis and hyaline membrane disease. *Am J Dis Child.* 1959;97:517.
3. Fujiwara T, Maeta H, Chida S, et al. Artificial surfactant therapy in hyaline-membrane disease. *Lancet.* 1980;1(8159):55–59.
4. Shennan AT, Dunn MS, Ohlsson A, et al. Abnormal pulmonary outcomes in premature infants: prediction from oxygen requirement in the neonatal period. *Pediatrics.* 1988;82:527–32.
5. Dunn MS, Shennan AT, Hoskins EM, et al. Two-year follow-up of infants enrolled in a randomized trial of surfactant replacement therapy for prevention of neonatal respiratory distress syndrome. *Pediatrics.* 1988; 82: 543–47.
6. Soll R, Özek E. Prophylactic animal derived surfactant extract for preventing morbidity and mortality in preterm infants. *Cochrane Database Syst. Rev.* 1997;(4):CD000511.
7. Schwartz RM, Luby AM, Scanlon JW, et al. Effect of surfactant on morbidity, mortality, and resource use in newborn infants weighing 500 to 1500 g. *N Engl J Med.* 1994;330:1476–80.

8. Jobe A, Ikegami M, Jacobs H, et al. Surfactant and pulmonary blood flow distributions following treatment of premature lambs with natural surfactant. *J Clinl Invest.* 1984;73:848–56.
9. Kendig JW, Notter RH, Cox C, et al. A comparison of surfactant as immediate prophylaxis and as rescue therapy in newborns of less than 30 weeks' gestation. *N Engl J Med.* 1991; 324:865–71.

11

Collaborative Quality Improvement to Promote Evidence-based Surfactant for Preterm Infants

A Cluster Randomized Trial

ASHRAF KHARRAT AND PRAKESH S. SHAH

"A multi-faceted collaborative improvement intervention . . . changed the behavior of neonatologists and promoted evidence based practice."
—HORBAR ET AL.[1]

Research Question: Does exposure to a multifaceted quality improvement (QI) intervention, versus standard care, improve timeliness of administration of surfactant and improve clinical outcomes to hospital discharge for infants 23 to 29 weeks' gestation?

Why Was This Study Done: Earlier surfactant administration was believed to reduce the risk of death and pneumothorax among preterm infants; however, lack of or delay in administration of this treatment was common at the time of this study.

Year Study Began: 2000

Year Study Published: 2004

Study Location: North America (114 centers)

Who Was Studied: NICUs participating in the Vermont Oxford Network

Who Was Excluded: Sites already participating in QI initiatives, sites where >50% very low birth weight infants are outborn, sites where >50% infants receive surfactant within 15 minutes of birth.

How Many Patients: 6039 infants, receiving care at 114 centers

Study Overview: This was a cluster RCT, with randomization at the level of the NICU (Figure 11.1).

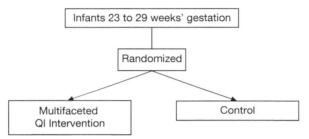

Figure 11.1 Study Overview

What Were the Interventions:
- NICUs randomized to the QI group received an intervention comprised of audit and feedback of surfactant practices from the previous 2 years, an interactive training workshop on how to conduct QI, and ongoing faculty support via conference calls and emails.
- NICUs randomized to the control group continued to receive center-specific reports, without any additional training or support.

How Long Was Follow-up: Hospital discharge

What Were the Endpoints:
Primary outcomes: Process of care measures (specifically various markers of speed of surfactant administration) and infant outcomes (mortality, pneumothorax).
Selected secondary outcomes: Common neonatal morbidities and co-interventions for preterm infants, including BPD, corticosteroid treatment for BPD, infection, IVH, and ROP.

Concerns Regarding Bias: Although cluster design might improve compliance with the intervention, a risk of performance bias remains, as knowledge of intervention sites receiving QI training may have impacted on care practices at control sites.

RESULTS

- Infants at intervention sites received surfactant almost one hour earlier than infants at control sites (median 21 minutes versus 78 minutes, adjusted hazard ratio 1.57, 95% CI 1.42 to 2.07, p <0.001).
- Infants at intervention sites had 5 times higher odds of receiving surfactant in the delivery room (adjusted odds ratio [aOR] 5.38, 95% CI 2.84 to 10.20) and 3 times lower odds of receiving surfactant treatment more than 2 hours after birth (aOR 0.35, 95% CI 0.24 to 0.53).
- Infants at intervention sites had lower odds of severe (grades 3–4) IVH compared with infants at control sites (aOR 0.70, 95% CI 0.56 to 0.87). The authors noted that a reduced risk of IVH is not known to be associated with earlier surfactant administration and suggested that other unmeasured changes in delivery room care may have occurred.
- There were no significant differences in other outcomes, including mortality, pneumothorax, and BPD.

Criticisms and Limitations: Cluster randomization plays a uniquely important role in QI studies, allowing a more natural implementation of interventions directed at groups of providers, who may find it difficult or impossible to randomly provide different care to individual patients. However, as a cluster randomized trial, this study loses some of the inherent benefits of trials randomized at the patient level, including the ability to evaluate treatment effects within sites and protection from covariate imbalances between sites.

This study saw robust results when providing centers with QI training to target the unique barriers in their centers. While very successful in improving process measures, this study demonstrated no impact on the primary outcome clinical measures of mortality and pneumothorax. This may be a power issue, given that the trial achieved a smaller increase in delivery room use of surfactant than anticipated; it is possible that clinical outcomes may have improved over a longer period of intervention.

Plans to encourage sustainability of the success in improving process measures were not specified in this study. It would be helpful to report ongoing maintenance of achieved improvement in process outcomes, as it is well known that the gains of QI interventions sometimes diminish after the active intervention period is over.

Other Relevant Studies and Information:
- This trial represented one of the first and largest QI trials in neonatal medicine.
- Other large-scale cluster RCTs of QI were subsequently undertaken and produced variable results. The National Institute of Child Health and Human Development Neonatal Research Network assessed the impact of QI training and benchmarking, and despite changes in respiratory practices, found similar rates of BPD.[2] The Evidence-based Practice for Improving Quality (EPIQ) study randomly assigned participating sites to target reduction of either nosocomial infections or BPD. It reported a 32% reduction in infections and a 15% reduction in BPD in respective QI study sites.[3]

Summary and Implications: This study explored the impact of multifaceted QI interventions on clinical practices in neonatology and demonstrated that a targeted QI strategy can improve process measures. Further, this study highlights that the cluster randomized trial is a feasible and appropriate method of assessing a large QI intervention. However, it also reminds us that improvement in process measures may not lead to improvement in clinical outcomes, and that a longer study period as well as careful consideration of balancing measures may be needed in the evaluation of QI activities.

A CONVERSATION WITH THE TRIALIST: JEFFREY HORBAR

Should process measures (as opposed to clinical events) be primary outcomes in future trials of QI, and if so, why?

Yes, when the causal pathway from process to outcome is well established. However, that conclusion is often fraught, as shown in our trail where early surfactant treatment was thought to lead to better outcomes. Although early surfactant treatment (process) was affected by the intervention, mortality and pneumothorax (outcomes) were not.

Why do you think so few other cluster trials of this sort in QI are done?

We were fortunate to have patient-level data from all hospitals as part of their participation in Vermont Oxford Network. This minimized additional data burden and allowed sites randomized to the control arm to participate without any added data collection burden.

Lack of incentives for control sites may be a barrier. Step wedge designs where everyone eventually receives the intervention is a potential solution.

This trial taught QI but allowed specific practices to be ascertained by the centers. It resulted in a change in process but not outcomes. How does one balance context (an essential element of QI) with heterogeneity in cluster trials of QI?

At Vermont Oxford Network we refer to practices as "potentially better" rather than "better" or "best" given our belief that evidence-based practices must be adapted and tested in the local context before they can be considered better or best. That is where QI and the Model for Improvement come in. Randomized trials are our strongest method for achieving unbiased estimates of the "average" effect size for an intervention, but weaker for determining in what contexts the intervention will be effective.

References

1. Horbar JD, Carpenter JH, Buzas J, et al. Collaborative quality improvement to promote evidence based surfactant for preterm infants: a cluster randomised trial. *BMJ*. 2004 Oct 28;329(7473):1004.
2. Walsh M, Laptook A, Kazzi SN, et al. A cluster-randomized trial of benchmarking and multimodal quality improvement to improve rates of survival free of bronchopulmonary dysplasia for infants with birth weights of less than 1250 grams. *Pediatrics*. 2007;119(5):876–90.
3. Lee SK, Aziz K, Singhal N, et al. Improving the quality of care for infants: a cluster randomized controlled trial. *CMAJ*. 2009;181(8):469–76.

Pressure-Regulated Volume Control Ventilation vs Synchronized Intermittent Mandatory Ventilation for Very Low Birth Weight Infants

ERIK A. JENSEN

"Pressure-regulated volume control (PRVC) does not provide any measurable advantage over [pressure-limited] synchronized intermittent mandatory ventilation (SIMV) in the treatment of premature newborns with respiratory distress syndrome. . . ."

—D'ANGIO ET AL.[1]

Research Question: Among infants weighing 500 to 1249 g at birth receiving invasive mechanical ventilation, does synchronized pressure-regulated volume control (PRVC) ventilation initiated within the first 6 hours after birth, compared with pressure-limited synchronized intermittent mandatory ventilation (SIMV), increase the proportion of infants who are alive and extubated at 14 days after birth?

Why Was This Study Done: Only 2 published trials (total number of participants = 110) that compared volume-targeted versus pressure-limited modes of invasive ventilation in newborns were available prior to the initiation of this trial.[2,3] The results of these 2 studies suggested that volume-targeted ventilation may shorten the duration of invasive ventilation and decrease the risk of IVH.

Year Study Began: 1998

Year Study Published: 2005

Study Location: United States (2 centers)

Who Was Studied: Infants within 6 hours after birth with birth weights of 500 to 1249 g and gestational ages of ≥24 weeks who were receiving invasive mechanical ventilation.

Who Was Excluded: No exclusion criteria were provided

How Many Patients: 212

Study Overview: This trial was a parallel-group, unmasked RCT (Figure 12.1).

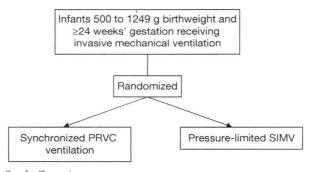

Figure 12.1 Study Overview

What Were the Interventions:
- Patients randomized to PRVC received an assist-control mode of ventilation that varies the delivered pressure to approximate a target inspiratory tidal volume.
- Patients randomized to SIMV received a pressure-limited mode of ventilation without supplemental pressure support.

Infants received their assigned mode of ventilation until extubation, death, or reaching pre-determined failure criteria. At these criteria, crossovers were allowed. Target PaO_2 (pressure of oxygen in arterial blood) and $PaCO_2$ (pressure of CO_2 in arterial blood) values were specified, but ventilator settings used to achieve these targets were determined by the clinical team.

How Long Was Follow-up: Hospital discharge

What Were the Endpoints:
Primary outcome: Composite outcome of survival and extubation within 14 days after birth.
Selected secondary outcomes: Measures of respiratory physiology recorded at 12 hours after birth, age at final extubation in survivors, survival without BPD, death prior to discharge, failure of the assigned mode of mechanical ventilation based on protocol-specified failure criteria, IVH, developmental abnormalities.

Concerns Regarding Bias: The study was at high risk for performance/ascertainment bias, as caregivers were not blinded to the intervention. Additionally, there was risk of bias given that
important secondary outcomes, such as developmental outcome, were only assessed at one center.

RESULTS

- No difference in the proportion of infants alive and extubated at 14 days after birth was detected between the PRVC group and the SIMV group (36.5% versus 40.7%; RR 0.90, 95% CI 0.64 to 1.26).
- Most secondary outcomes were similar between the 2 treatment groups. At 12 hours after birth, infants assigned to SIMV as compared with PRVC received significantly higher mean tidal volumes (17.8 versus 14.1 mL/kg; mean difference [MD]) –3.5, 95% CI –5.0 to –2.0. Notably, these values were measured at the ventilator without correction for dead space contributed by the respiratory circuit) and higher mean peak inspiratory pressures (14.0 versus 12.7 cm H_2O; MD –1.4, 95% CI –2.1 to –0.6), but lower ventilator rates (30 versus 40 breaths/min; MD 9, 95% CI 7 to 12). Minute ventilation recorded at 12 hours after birth was similar between the treatment groups.
- Rates of final extubation (i.e., no further invasive mechanical ventilation) by 14 days after birth were significantly lower among infants assigned to PRVC than SIMV (19.2% versus 33.3%; RR 0.58, 95% CI 0.36 to 0.93). More infants assigned to the SIMV group than to the PRVC group failed the assigned ventilator mode (33.3% versus 20.2%; RR 0.61, 95% CI 0.38 to 0.97).
- No difference in the rates of survival without BPD were detected between the PRVC group and the SIMV group (63.5% versus 57.1%; RR 0.83, 95% CI 0.55 to 1.27).

Criticisms and Limitations: This trial provided important data to compare outcomes between infants randomized to receive PRVC—then a new mode of volume-targeted mode of ventilation—versus SIMV—a pressure-limited mode of ventilation. These results factored heavily into meta-analyses comparing volume versus pressure-control modes of ventilation.[2] Nonetheless, limitations of the trial affect interpretation and application of the study findings.

First, the primary trial outcome, the composite of survival up to and extubation at 14 days of age, was a short-term endpoint. The study was powered to detect an arguably implausible difference in this outcome (20% absolute differences in rates); and was underpowered to measure significant differences in the more clinically relevant outcomes of BPD and neurodevelopment. Second, although the trial protocol specified target arterial PaO_2 and $PaCO_2$ levels, recommended ventilator settings were not provided. This may produce significant within-arm heterogeneity in ventilator management and hinder clinicians' ability to replicate the trial therapy. Third, pressure support levels were placed at 0 cm H_2O in the infants randomized to receive SIMV. The authors indicate this approach was taken to "maximize the difference in the number of supported breaths between SIMV and PRVC." However, imbalance in the proportion of ventilator-supported breaths may have led to important physiologic differences between infants in the 2 trial arms. These limitations complicate assessment of the risks and benefits of volume compared with pressure-control modes of invasive ventilation. This approach of zero pressure support in SIMV is also inconsistent with how the mode of ventilation is often used. Lastly, clinicians were not masked to the assigned ventilator mode. This limitation is commonplace in trials of respiratory support modalities, which is why criteria for extubation readiness and treatment failure are often prespecified. Despite these attempted safeguards, alternative treatment choices made by clinicians may introduce bias, as was possible in this trial where rates of ventilator failure attributed to "attending neonatologist's discretion" were higher (although not statistically different) in the SIMV group (20.3%) compared with the PRVC group (12.5%).

Other Relevant Studies and Information:
- A 2017 Cochrane Review included the results from 16 parallel-group RCTs (977 infants) that compared outcomes among infants treated with a volume-targeted versus pressure-limited modes of mechanical ventilation.[4] This meta-analysis demonstrated that volume-targeted ventilation reduced the risk of the composite outcome of death or BPD, pneumothorax, mean days of mechanical ventilation, hypocarbia, grade 3 or 4 IVH, and periventricular leukomalacia. Overall quality of the evidence was low to moderate, owing to lack of masking, as well as design issues in other included trials. The D'Angio trial provided the

largest proportion of weight for the composite outcome of death or
BPD.
- Volume-targeted ventilation is now the preferred approach to the
  management of preterm infants with respiratory distress syndrome who
  are treated with conventional mechanical ventilation.[5]

Summary and Implications: This trial was among the first RCTs to compare synchronized volume-targeted mechanical ventilation to pressure-limited mechanical ventilation in preterm infants. Although this trial showed similar outcomes between the 2 modes of ventilation, its large contribution in meta-analyses led to practice change among NICUs towards volume-targeted ventilation.

A CONVERSATION WITH THE TRIALIST: CARL D'ANGIO

Given the results of your study and the Cochrane meta-analysis, practice has shifted such that over one-half of units in an international survey were using volume ventilation; that survey also showed significant variation in practice and suggested further trials to establish.[1] As the author of the study carrying the greatest weight, what further studies are needed, and is there a need for comparison to less conventional approaches to ventilation?

Ventilation is an area in which technology tends to run ahead of evidence. The Cochrane meta-analysis includes studies from 20–25 years ago, when the sophistication of ventilators was very different than today's. The capability for providing true volume or volume-targeted ventilation is superior to what was available when our study was performed. This points to the continued need of study of new modes that have not been fully tested among infants before they become available. Studies comparing "traditional" volume and pressure modes to less conventional modes are also necessary as these modes arise.

As I tell my trainees, we have gotten much better at ventilation in the last 25 years, but don't really know why. More sophisticated sensors and software are doubtless part of the explanation, but it has been difficult to prove this point with single studies comparing modes. It is likely that our success has been the result of sequential small improvements, some of which never meet the statistical requirement for superiority, that have combined to improve our approach.

1. Klingenberg C, Wheeler KI, Owen LS, et al. An international survey of volume-targeted neonatal ventilation. *Arch Dis Child Fetal Neonatal Ed.* 2011;96(2):F146–8.

References

1. D'Angio CT, Chess PR, Kovacs SJ, et al. Pressure-regulated volume control ventilation vs synchronized intermittent mandatory ventilation for very low-birth-weight infants: a randomized controlled trial. *Arch Pediatr Adolesc Med.* 2005;159(9):868–75.
2. Piotrowski A, Sobala W, Kawczyński P. Patient-initiated, pressure-regulated, volume-controlled ventilation compared with intermittent mandatory ventilation in neonates: a prospective, randomised study. *Intensive Care Med.* 1997;23(9):975–81.
3. Sinha SK, Donn SM, Gavey J, et al. Randomised trial of volume controlled versus time cycled, pressure limited ventilation in preterm infants with respiratory distress syndrome. *Arch Dis Child Fetal Neonatal Ed.* 1997;77(3):F202–5.
4. Klingenberg C, Wheeler KI, McCallion N, et al. Volume-targeted versus pressure-limited ventilation in neonates. *Cochrane Database Syst Rev.* 2017;10(10):CD003666.
5. Sweet DG, Carnielli V, Greisen G, et al. European Consensus Guidelines on the Management of Respiratory Distress Syndrome - 2019 Update. *Neonatology.* 2019;115(4):432–50.

13

Long-term Effects of Caffeine Therapy for Apnea of Prematurity

The CAP Trial

DIRK BASSLER

"The present results, showing that caffeine significantly improved survival without neurodevelopmental disability at a corrected age of 18 to 21 months, provide strong evidence that the overall benefits of methylxanthine therapy as used in this trial outweigh any potential risks up to 2 years after very preterm birth."

—SCHMIDT ET AL.[1]

Research Question: Among infants with birth weights of 500 to 1250 g, does caffeine therapy for apnea of prematurity (AoP) alter the rate of survival without neurodevelopmental disability at 18 to 21 months' CA?

Why Was This Study Done: At the time of this trial, caffeine was a long-accepted treatment for AoP and one of the most frequently used medications in the NICU. However, this was based on scant evidence, and reasonable doubt had emerged on strong biological grounds among the neonatal community about its safety and long-term effects.

Year Study Began: 1999

Year Study Published: 2007

Study Location: Canada, Australia, The Netherlands, Israel, United States, United Kingdom, Sweden, Switzerland, Germany

Who Was Studied: Infants with a birth weight of 500 to 1250 g if their clinicians considered them as candidates for caffeine therapy during the first 10 days of life.

Who Was Excluded: Infants with dysmorphic features or congenital abnormalities likely to affect life expectancy or neurologic development, and those previously treated with a methylxanthine.

How Many Patients: 2006

Study Overview: The CAP (Caffeine for Apnea of Prematurity) trial was a parallel-group, masked RCT (Figure 13.1).

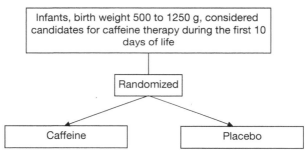

Figure 13.1 Study Overview

What Were the Interventions:
- Infants randomized to the caffeine group received an intravenous (IV) loading dose of caffeine 20 mg/kg. This was followed by a daily maintenance dose of 5 mg/kg. If apneas persisted, the daily maintenance dose could be increased to a maximum of 10 mg/kg. The maintenance doses were adjusted weekly for changes in body weight and could be given orally once an infant tolerated full enteral feedings.
- Infants randomized to the placebo group received doses of equivalent volumes of normal saline.

How Long Was Follow-up: 18 to 21 months' CA

What Were the Endpoints:
Primary outcome: Composite outcome of death, cerebral palsy, cognitive delay, deafness, or blindness.

Selected secondary outcomes: Individual components of the primary outcome, growth parameters, ROP.

Concerns Regarding Bias: The study was at overall low risk of bias.

RESULTS

- Caffeine was superior to placebo for the primary composite outcome of death or neurodevelopmental disability at 18–21 months' CA (adjusted odds ratio [aOR] for center 0.77, 95% CI 0.64 to 0.93, p = 0.008).
- Treatment with caffeine reduced the incidence of cerebral palsy (aOR 0.58, 95% CI, 0.39 to 0.87, p = 0.009) and cognitive delay (aOR 0.81, 95% CI 0.66 to 0.99, p = 0.04).
- There were no differences in the rates of death, deafness, and blindness; nor were there differences in the mean percentiles for height, weight, and head circumference.
- Post hoc analysis showed a decrease in severe ROP with caffeine therapy (aOR 0.61, 95% CI 0.42 to 0.89, p = 0.01).
- Evaluation of 6 explanatory variables (postmenstrual ages at last use of 3 levels of respiratory support, use of postnatal corticosteroids, PDA surgery, and BPD) suggested that together they explained 55% of the observed benefit of caffeine therapy on survival without neurodevelopmental disability.

Criticisms and Limitations: This trial has been heralded as among the most rigorous and influential in the field.[2] A few considerations could be made for its interpretation.

The authors chose a pragmatic approach by not measuring the immediate known effects of caffeine on apnea itself, on plausible grounds that apnea is difficult to measure reliably whether by respiratory monitoring or by nursing reports. Furthermore, they enrolled a broad range of patients, who might be considered for treatment. They focused on neurodevelopmental assessment, although they chose a rather early time point of 2 years for assessment. The Bayley Scales may not be the ideal instrument to reveal differences at this early stage. However, the CAP trial was able to demonstrate statistically and clinically important differences already at 18–21 months' CA, and subsequent follow-up studies of this cohort confirmed the positive effect of caffeine.

If mortality had differed between the groups (in either direction), the interpretation of the primary composite outcome could have been problematic. For example, imagine a scenario where caffeine increased mortality but decreased neurodevelopmental impairment. However, the CAP trial did not show any difference in mortality between the 2 groups, which makes the interpretation of the results straightforward.

Other Relevant Studies and Information:
- Earlier reporting suggested by the Data and Safety Monitoring Board, of this cohort showed that caffeine therapy reduced the incidence of BPD (36.3% versus 46.9%; aOR 0.63, 95% CI 0.52 to 0.76, p <0.001).[3] Pulmonary function additionally appeared improved in caffeine-treated patients at 11 year follow-up.[4]
- Subsequent follow-up of this cohort at 5 years demonstrated no difference in the composite outcome of death or disability.[5] However, secondary measures of motor impairment were improved by caffeine at 5 years, and again at 11 years of age.[6]
- Benefits of caffeine appeared similar across clinical indications for treatment.[7]
- Timing of initiation of caffeine, its indications, and dose ranges are less well studied and remain, at least partly, controversial.[8,9]

Summary and Implications: The CAP trial is a large and rigorous pragmatic trial that demonstrated that caffeine improves survival without neurodevelopmental disability at 18 to 21 months' CA. It provides strong evidence that the overall benefits of caffeine therapy as used in this trial outweigh potential risks, and led to widespread adoption and standardization of this treatment.

A CONVERSATION WITH THE TRIALIST: BARBARA SCHMIDT

Your study employed thoughtful composite endpoints to assess neurodevelopment. Could you comment on the use of composite endpoints in neonatal trials, including the decision to include death as a component?

The primary outcome of the CAP trial at 18 to 21 months was a composite of death, cerebral palsy, cognitive delay, deafness, or blindness. We chose this main endpoint because it was relevant, reproducible, and potentially responsive to the trial intervention. Caffeine reduced this outcome.

A carefully designed composite outcome has many advantages. It avoids the arbitrary choice of a single outcome when several are similarly important, reduces problems of multiple testing, and accounts for competing risks. A composite endpoint may also estimate "net clinical benefit" if efficacy and safety outcomes are combined.

Criticisms have focused on flaws in the choice of components, incomplete reporting of the results for each of the components, and misinterpretation of composite outcomes by consumers of the research. All these problems are largely preventable by careful study design, adequate reporting of the composite and its components, and education of the end users of the trial reports.

It has been argued that death should not be combined with disability in a composite outcome because death trumps all other outcomes in importance for parents. However, judgements about the importance of death vs disability are subjective and influenced by cultural backgrounds and religious beliefs. There is no agreement among either clinicians or parents of sick and preterm infants whether grieving for a lost baby is always worse than caring for a disabled child.

Even critics who dispute that death and disability can ever be of similar importance must acknowledge that death in many of our neonatal trial populations is frequent enough to be a competing risk we simply cannot ignore in our research. In fact, death is not the only competing risk in the composite of death or disability as we defined it for the CAP trial. Cognition may be impossible to assess in survivors with physical impairments. To avoid attrition bias, it is therefore wise to combine cognition with physical impairments in a composite long-term outcome for neonatal trials of high-risk infants.

References

1. Schmidt B, Roberts RS, Davis P, et al.; Caffeine for Apnea of Prematurity Trial Group. Long-term effects of caffeine therapy for apnea of prematurity. *N Engl J Med.* 2007;357:1893–902.

2. Kreutzer K, Bassler D. Caffeine for apnea of prematurity: a neonatal success story. *Neonatology.* 2014;105(4):332–6.

3. Schmidt B, Roberts R, Davis P, et al. Caffeine therapy for apnea of prematurity. *N Engl J Med.* 2006;354(20):2112–21.

4. Doyle J, Ranganathan S, Cheong J. Neonatal caffeine treatment and respiratory function at 11 years in children under 1,251 g at birth. *Am J Respir Crit Care Med.* 2017;196(10):1318–24.

5. Schmidt B, Anderson P, Doyle L, et al. Survival without disability to age 5 years after neonatal caffeine therapy for apnea of prematurity. *J Am Med Assoc.* 2012;307:275–82.

6. Schmidt B, Roberts R, Anderson P, et al. Academic performance, motor function, and behavior 11 years after neonatal caffeine citrate therapy for apnea of prematurity: an 11-year follow-up of the CAP randomized clinical trial. *JAMA Pediatr.* 2017;171(6):564–72.

7. Davis PG, Schmidt B, Roberts RS, et al.; Caffeine for Apnea of Prematurity Trial Group. Caffeine for Apnea of Prematurity trial: benefits may vary in subgroups. *J Pediatr.* 2010 Mar;156(3):382–7.
8. Sweet DG, Carnielli V, Greisen G, et al. European consensus guidelines on the management of respiratory distress syndrome – 2019 update. *Neonatology.* 2019;115:432–50.
9. Rodgers A, Singh C. Specialist neonatal respiratory care for babies born preterm (NICE guideline 124,): a review. *Arch Dis Child Educ Pract Ed.* 2020. https://www.nice.org.uk/guidance/ng124.

14

Outcome at Two Years of Age of Infants From the DART Study

A Multicenter, International, Randomized Controlled Trial of Low-Dose Dexamethasone

The DART Trial

WES ONLAND AND ANTON H. VAN KAAM

"Although this trial was not able to provide definitive evidence on the long-term effects of low-dose dexamethasone after the first week of life in chronically ventilator-dependent infants, our data indicate no strong association with long-term morbidity."

—DOYLE ET AL.[1]

Research Question: Does a tapering low-dose dexamethasone regimen, versus placebo, initiated after the first week of life in ventilator-dependent, preterm infants impact long-term neurodevelopmental outcome at 2 years corrected age (CA)?

Why Was This Study Done: At the time of this trial, the various tradeoffs of dexamethasone—in particular that between ease of extubation and long-term neurodevelopmental outcomes—were quite uncertain. The aim of DART (Dexamethasone: A Randomized Trial) was to examine the effects of low-dose dexamethasone on long-term rates of survival free of major neurologic disability.

Year Study Began: 2000

Year Study Published: 2007

Study Location: Australia, New Zealand, Canada (11 centers total)

Who Was Studied: Extremely preterm (<28 weeks' gestation) or extremely low birth weight (ELBW; <1000 g) infants who were ventilator-dependent after the first week of life.

Who Was Excluded: Infants with congenital neurologic defects or other disorders, such as chromosomal anomalies, likely to cause substantial long-term neurologic deficits.

How Many Patients: 70. Of note, the DART study had a target sample size of 814, to detect an improvement in survival free of major neurosensory disability from 50% to 60%. However, enrollment had to be abandoned after 2 years of recruitment because of increasing lack of clinician equipoise and difficulty with recruitment following various professional and American Academy of Pediatrics (AAP) statements.

In a 2002 letter to *Pediatrics,* study principal investigator Lex Doyle wrote about the professional guidance to limit postnatal use of systemic dexamethasone for the prevention or treatment of BPD to RCTs, "In an apparent paradox, since the joint statement by AAP and the Canadian Paediatric Society in February, recruitment has dropped, not increased. Moreover, the uncertainty has not been translated into new centers wanting to join the study."[2]

Study Overview: The DART trial was a parallel-group, masked RCT (Figure 14.1).

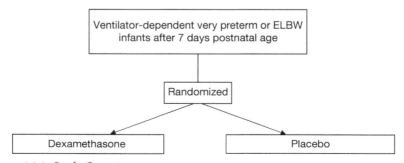

Figure 14.1 Study Overview

What Were the Interventions:
- Patients randomized to the dexamethasone group received twice-daily doses of a 10-day tapering course of dexamethasone sodium phosphate (0.15 mg/kg per day for 3 days, 0.10 mg/kg per day for 3 days, 0.05 mg/kg per day for 2 days, and 0.02 mg/kg per day for 2 days; cumulative dose of 0.89 mg/kg).
- Patients randomized to the placebo group received saline in equivalent volume and frequency.

How Long Was Follow-up: 2 years CA

What Were the Endpoints:
Primary outcome: Composite outcome of survival free of major neurosensory disability at 2 years CA. Major neurosensory disability was defined as having cerebral palsy (CP), blindness, deafness, or a mental developmental index score <85 of the Bayley Scales of Infant Development-Second Edition (BSID-II).
Selected secondary outcomes: Hospital readmissions, duration of home oxygen therapy, growth, any serious adverse events.

Concerns Regarding Bias: The study was at overall low risk of bias. Although the study was terminated early, this was independent of the trial findings.

RESULTS

- No difference in the composite outcome of death or major neurosensory disability was detected (dexamethasone 45.7% versus placebo 42.9%; RR 1.07, 95% CI 0.63 to 1.80).
- No differences were found in any of the components of the composite primary outcome, and the separate components of the outcome neurosensory disability, such as CP, blindness, and deafness. Anthropometric outcomes at 2 years CA (blood pressure, hospital readmission, and duration of home oxygen therapy) were also not different between the 2 groups.

Criticisms and Limitations: Trial recruitment was ended after 2.5 years with less than 10% of the intended number of participants randomized. The statistical power of this trial is therefore very low, and the ability to draw conclusions from this trial on administration of low-dose dexamethasone after the first week of life to mechanically ventilated extremely preterm infants at risk for neurodevelopmental impairment (NDI) is limited. The tragedy of this trial was the intense professional criticism that prematurely ended a trial that could have yielded enormous clarification for the community.

The timing and cumulative dosage regimen investigated in the DART trial, as well as the use of open-label corticosteroid administration, are worth discussing. Since RCTs investigating early dexamethasone administration during the first week of life have shown an increased risk of NDI, initiating therapy only after 7 days of life seems justified.[3,4] However, subgroup and meta-regression analyses of all placebo-controlled dexamethasone trials after the first week of life show that the cumulative dexamethasone dose, the timing of initiating therapy, and the rate of open-label use modify long-term pulmonary and neurodevelopmental outcomes.[4-7] Most infants included in the DART trial started the low-dose dexamethasone regimen in the fourth week of life, which might have hampered the beneficial effect of dexamethasone.[6] Forty percent of infants in the placebo group were treated with open-label dexamethasone, which might have diluted potential benefit or harm from dexamethasone treatment.[7]

Other Relevant Studies and Information:
- In 2006, the outcomes to hospital discharge of the DART trial were reported, such as BPD, failure to extubate, and various adverse outcomes.[8] None of the reported outcomes differed between the 2 groups, except the number of infants with failure to extubate. In the group allocated to dexamethasone treatment, more infants were extubated successfully after 10 days of treatment (60%) than in the placebo group (12%) (p <0.01).[8]
- The results of the DART trial have contributed to the revised statement of the American Academy of Pediatrics (AAP) that low-dose dexamethasone therapy may facilitate extubation and decrease the incidence of short- and long-term adverse effects observed with higher doses of dexamethasone, but that additional sufficiently powered RCTs are needed.[9]
- The Cochrane review on systemic postnatal corticosteroid treatment after the first week of life concluded that treatment reduces the risks of mortality and BPD, without evidence of increased NDI. However, the methodological quality and number of studies with long-term outcomes is limited.[10]

Summary and Implications: The 2-year outcomes of the DART trial showed no differences in death or major neurosensory disability between ventilated extremely preterm infants treated with low-dose dexamethasone therapy, initiated after the first week, compared with placebo. However, recruitment had to be abandoned because collective equipoise was lost soon after the trial was launched, and the results are therefore inconclusive. The debate regarding the use of corticosteroids in preterm infants, including the right indication, drug, optimal timing, and dosage, continues. Although imprecise, the results of this trial, showing no increased risk in adverse long-term neurodevelopmental outcomes, led to a practice change of prescribing low-dose dexamethasone to facilitate weaning and extubation in mechanically ventilated preterm infants.

A CONVERSATION WITH THE TRIALIST: LEX DOYLE

Given that a large number of families were not approached at physician's request and that a sizeable number of infants were treated with steroids outside the trial, can you tell us what happened to collective equipoise after you launched DART?

DART was conceived and conducted in difficult times. Equipoise was changing rapidly. To conduct the study we needed to recruit not only individual clinicians who were still in equipoise, but individual units where all clinicians were in equipoise.

Although individual clinicians and their units ultimately joined the study, they were not in equipoise concerning all babies. Although ideally we would have liked to insist on no open-label corticosteroids at all, we could not run such a study because no one would have joined; clinicians were too "steroid-dependent." I would not describe the clinicians' behaviour as irrational—they were using their clinical judgement and acting in the best interests of their babies and their families at the time.

Would the sabotage of the DART trial still be possible nowadays?

The largest difference today compared with 20 years ago is that the rate of treatment with systemic corticosteroids to prevent or treat BPD has [significantly decreased][1] and is unlikely to fluctuate dramatically over the next few years. Despite [the concerns], clinicians continue to prescribe corticosteroids for almost 1 out of every 10 very low birth weight infants.[1]

The biggest issue that dogged the DART study still exists today: that of open-label corticosteroids. There have been other RCTS of systemic corticosteroids since DART, and all of them have allowed open-label treatment with corticosteroids, including 3 of the most recent and largest RCTS.[2–4]

While we continue to allow "rescue" treatment, the true effects of systemic corticosteroids within RCTS will continue to be masked. However, an open-label-free RCT is unlikely to be permitted on ethical grounds, given the continued high rate of "steroid-dependency" we see in clinical practice today.

1. Walsch MC, Yao Q, Horbar JD, et al. Changes in the use of postnatal steroids for bronchopulmonary dysplasia in 3 large neonatal networks. *Pediatrics.* 2006;118(5):e1328–35.
2. Baud O, Maury L, Lebail F, et al. Effect of early low-dose hydrocortisone on survival without bronchopulmonary dysplasia in extremely preterm infants (PREMILOC): a double-blind, placebo-controlled, multicentre, randomised trial. *Lancet* 2016; 387(10030):1827–36.
3. Onland W, Cools F, Kroon A, et al. Effect of hydrocortisone therapy initiated 7 to 14 days after birth on mortality or bronchopulmonary dysplasia among very preterm infants receiving mechanical ventilation: a randomized clinical trial. *JAMA* 2019; 321(4):354–63.
4. Watterberg KL, Walsh MC, Li L, et al. Hydrocortisone to improve survival without bronchopulmonary dysplasia. *N Engl J Med* 2022; 386(12):1121–31.

References

1. Doyle LW, Davis PG, Morley CJ, et al.; DART Study Investigators. Outcome at 2 Years of Age of Infants From the DART Study: A Multicenter, International, Randomized, Controlled Trial of Low-Dose Dexamethasone. *Pediatrics.* 2007;119(4):716–21.
2. Doyle L, Davis P, Morley C. Effect of AAP Statement regarding postnatal corticosteroids on ongoing and future randomized, controlled trials. Letter to the Editor. *Pediatrics.* 2002;110(5):1032–3.
3. Doyle LW, Cheong JL, Hay S, et al. Early (<7 days) systemic postnatal corticosteroids for prevention of bronchopulmonary dysplasia in preterm infants. *Cochrane Database Syst Rev.* 2021;10:CD001146.
4. Doyle LW, Halliday HL, Ehrencranz RA, et al. Impact of postnatal systemic corticosteroids on mortality and cerebral palsy in preterm infants: effect modification by risk for chronic lung disease. *Pediatrics.* 2005;115(3):655–61.
5. Onland W, De Jaegere AP, Offringa M, et al. Systemic corticosteroid regimens for prevention of bronchopulmonary dysplasia in preterm infants. *Cochrane Database Syst Rev.* 2017;1:CD010941.
6. Onland W, Offringa M, De Jaegere AP, et al. Finding the optimal postnatal dexamethasone regimen for preterm infants at risk of bronchopulmonary dysplasia: a systematic review of placebo-controlled trials. *Pediatrics.* 2009;123(1):367–77.
7. Onland W, van Kaam AH, De Jaegere AP, et al. Open-label glucocorticoids modulate dexamethasone trial results in preterm infants. *Pediatrics.* 2010;126(4):e954–e64.
8. Doyle LW, Davis PG, Morley CJ, et al. Low-dose dexamethasone facilitates extubation among chronically ventilator-dependent infants: a multicenter, international, randomized, controlled trial. *Pediatrics.* 2006;117(1):75–83.
9. Watterberg KL. Policy statement--postnatal corticosteroids to prevent or treat bronchopulmonary dysplasia. *Pediatrics.* 2010;126(4):800–8.
10. Doyle LW, Cheong JL, Hay S, et al. Late (≥7 days) systemic postnatal corticosteroids for prevention of bronchopulmonary dysplasia in preterm infants. *Cochrane Database Syst Rev.* 2021;11:CD001145.

15

Early CPAP Versus Surfactant in Extremely Preterm Infants

The SUPPORT Trial

BRETT J. MANLEY

> "The results of this study support consideration of CPAP as an alternative to intubation and surfactant in [extremely] preterm infants."
> —SUPPORT STUDY GROUP[1]

Research Question: In extremely preterm infants born 24 to 27 weeks' gestation, does early continuous positive airway pressure (CPAP) treatment, compared with routine endotracheal intubation and surfactant therapy, reduce the composite outcome of death or BPD at 36 weeks' PMA?

Why Was This Study Done: Although earlier trials of prophylactic surfactant showed promising outcomes, observational evidence suggested that that earlier use of CPAP and selective surfactant could safely decrease the need for mechanical ventilation.

Year Study Began: 2005

Year Study Published: 2010

Study Location: United States (>20 centers within the Neonatal Research Network, NICHD)

Who Was Studied: Extremely preterm infants, born at 24 to 27 weeks' gestation

Who Was Excluded: Known malformations, or decision made not to provide full resuscitation

How Many Patients: 1316

Study Overview: The SUPPORT (Surfactant, Positive Pressure, and Oxygenation Randomized Trial) trial was an unmasked RCT with a 2-by-2 factorial design: infants were randomized before birth to either planned stabilization on CPAP or routine intubation in the delivery room; and to 2 different oxygen saturation target ranges upon NICU admission (Figure 15.1). (Nota bene: the results of the oxygen targeting arm of the trial are reported in Chapter 16.)

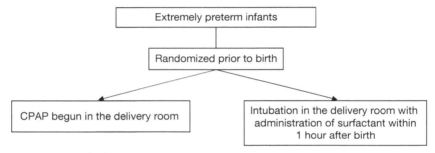

Figure 15.1 Study Overview

What Were the Interventions:
- Infants randomized to the CPAP group received CPAP in the delivery room, continuing until the infant's admission to the neonatal intensive care unit (NICU). Infants in this group who required intubation for resuscitation as per Neonatal Resuscitation Program guidelines were given surfactant within 1 hour after birth. This arm allowed later intubation for respiratory support in the NICU, provided standard criteria were met, with subsequent extubation guided by specified clinical criteria.
- Infants randomized to the surfactant group were intubated in the delivery room and received surfactant within 1 hour after birth, with continued mechanical ventilation thereafter. The infants were subsequently extubated according to specific criteria that differed from those in the CPAP group (with a threshold for extubation at lower respiratory support levels in the surfactant group).

How Long Was Follow-up: Hospital discharge

What Were the Endpoints:
Primary outcome: Composite outcome of death or BPD at 36 weeks' PMA.
Selected secondary outcomes: Pneumothorax, IVH, ROP.

Concerns Regarding Bias: The trial was at high risk for performance/detection bias, as caregivers were not blinded to the intervention.

RESULTS

- After adjustment for gestational age, center, and familial clustering, the rate of the primary outcome of death or BPD did not differ between the 2 groups (CPAP 47.8% versus intubation 51.0%; RR 0.95, 95% CI 0.85 to 1.05, $p = 0.30$).
- More infants in the CPAP group were alive and not receiving mechanical ventilation by day 7 (55.3% versus 48.8%; RR 1.14, 95% CI 1.03 to 1.25, $p = 0.01$), and infants in the CPAP group had fewer days of ventilation (adjusted mean 24.8 versus 27.7; mean difference –3.0, 95% CI –5.6 to –0.3, $p = 0.03$).
- There were no significant differences in the rates of common complications in extremely preterm infants, including pneumothorax, IVH, and ROP.

Criticisms and Limitations: Infants were randomized *before* birth, and around one-third of infants in the CPAP group subsequently required intubation during resuscitation. For infants intubated in the delivery room, only 41% in the CPAP group and 51% in the surfactant group received surfactant in the delivery room. Both of these factors might have obscured some true differences in outcomes between the groups.

Several considerations regarding generalizability are worth noting. Generalizability may have been impacted by the very high receipt of corticosteroids in enrolled mothers.[2] Additionally, infants born at a gestational age of <24 weeks' were not included, as the results of a pilot trial had shown that all such infants required intubation in the delivery room.[3] Thus, as practices change in favor of noninvasive respiratory management, it is difficult to extrapolate the results of the SUPPORT trial to the most immature infants. The mean gestation of infants included in this trial was 26 weeks; however, post hoc stratified analysis of the most immature infants (24 to 25 weeks' gestation) suggested benefit from stabilization on CPAP.

Similarly changes in preferences for application of CPAP may also affect either internal or external validity. These changes include differences in the CPAP pressures applied, the different thresholds for intubation, or the use of less invasive surfactant administration techniques.

Other Relevant Studies and Information:
- The international, multicenter "COIN" trial,[4] published prior to SUPPORT, randomized 610 extremely preterm infants to CPAP or intubation and ventilation at 5 minutes after birth (in contrast to SUPPORT which randomized infants *prior* to birth). At 36 weeks' PMA, 33.9% of the CPAP group and 38.9% of the intubation group had died or had BPD ($p = 0.19$).
- Other investigators have investigated the use of early CPAP in the delivery room. COIN and Sandri et al.[5] enrolled infants only after they proved needing intubation. The Dunn trial[6] of the Vermont Oxford Network looked at similar strategies for prophylactic surfactant versus CPAP, but had a third arm of intubation, surfactant treatment, and expedient extubation.
- A subsequent meta-analysis of these 4 RCTs (a total of 2782 very preterm infants) compared nasal CPAP in the delivery room with routine intubation and found a significant benefit for the combined outcome of death or BPD at 36 weeks' PMA (RR 0.90; 95% CI 0.83 to 0.98).[7]
- Guidelines have supported use of early CPAP and selective surfactant administration, as an alternative to routine intubation with prophylactic early surfactant.[8,9]
- While this trial supports the use of CPAP, it does not inform us on many nuances of the technology. The optimal CPAP pressure or interface remains to be determined.[10]
- Other innovative approaches to treatment may alter our application of the findings of SUPPORT. For example, the OptiMIST-A trial has recently shown that the use of a less invasive surfactant administration (LISA) technique in spontaneously breathing extremely preterm infants on CPAP reduces the incidence of BPD,[11] and multiple studies have demonstrated the feasibility of minimally or less-invasive surfactant administration, with the potential benefit of earlier surfactant administration to infants on CPAP.[12]

Summary and Implications: This trial is one of several that has shown some benefit for the use of CPAP as opposed to routine intubation in the delivery room and beyond, which subsequently became standard practice in many parts of the world. Further research will elucidate how other technologies, including nuances to the application of CPAP and earlier surfactant via less-invasive administration, may further influence our choices of care.

A CONVERSATION WITH THE TRIALIST: NEIL FINER

Are there aspects of trial design unrelated to CPAP that you think may have influenced outcome?

The first issue here is to discuss the impact of antenatal consent. We did review the outcomes of the infants in the trial and compared that to the outcomes of infants who were not consented or approached and found that the enrolled infants were advantaged in a number of ways.—These included better maternal antenatal care and more often exposed to antenatal steroids, better educated mothers, etc. . . . Enrolled infants had significantly lower rates of death before discharge, severe IVH/PVL, death/severe IVH/PVL [periventricular leukomalacia], and bronchopulmonary dysplasia in comparison with eligible, but not enrolled infants.

Can you comment on the unique considerations of testing technology in a changing landscape, e.g., differences in applied CPAP pressures/devices/ interfaces?

Certainly there has been a number of newer approaches that need further testing. Among these the most promising is LISA, not well studied in the USA but more widely practiced in Europe. Other approaches including aerosolization of surfactant have yet to be proven effective in the ELBW [extremely low birth weight] infant. There are newer interfaces for CPAP and the use of hi flow cannula that may be a substitute for direct CPAP, but further studies are required especially for the ELBW infant. Others are studying early lung recruitment in the delivery room using incrementally higher airway pressures.

References

1. SUPPORT Study Group of the Eunice Kennedy Shriver NICHD Neonatal Research Network, Finer NN, Carlo WA, et al. Early CPAP versus surfactant in extremely preterm infants. *N Engl J Med*. 2010;362(21):1970–9.
2. Rich WD, Auten KJ, Gantz MG, et al; National Institute of Child Health and Human Development Neonatal Research Network. Antenatal consent in the SUPPORT trial: challenges, costs, and representative enrollment. *Pediatrics*. 2010 Jul;126(1):e215–21.

3. Finer NN, Carlo WA, Duara S, et al.; National Institute of Child Health and Human Development Neonatal Research Network. Delivery room continuous positive airway pressure/positive end-expiratory pressure in extremely low birth weight infants: a feasibility trial. *Pediatrics*. 2004 Sep;114(3):651–7.
4. Morley CJ, Davis PG, Doyle LW, et al. Nasal CPAP or intubation at birth for very preterm infants. *N Engl J Med*. 2008;358(7):700–8.
5. Sandri F, Plavka R, Ancora G, et al. Prophylactic or early selective surfactant combined with nCPAP in very preterm infants. *Pediatrics*. 2010;125(6):e1402–9.
6. Dunn MS, Kaempf J, de Klerk A, et al. Randomized trial comparing 3 approaches to the initial respiratory management of preterm neonates. *Pediatrics*. 2011;128(5):e1069–76.
7. Schmolzer GM, Kumar M, Pichler G, et al. Non-invasive versus invasive respiratory support in preterm infants at birth: systematic review and meta-analysis. *BMJ*. 2013;347:f5980.
8. Committee on Fetus and Newborn. Policy statement: respiratory support in preterm infants at birth. *Pediatrics*. 2014;133(1):171–4.
9. Sweet DG, Carnielli V, Greisen G, et al. European consensus guidelines on the management of respiratory distress syndrome - 2019 update. *Neonatology*. 2019;115(4):432–4.
10. Bamat N, Fierro J, Mukerji A, et al. Nasal continuous positive airway pressure levels for the prevention of morbidity and mortality in preterm infants. *Cochrane Database Syst Rev*. 2021;(11):CD012778.
11. Dargaville PA, Kamlin COF, Orsini F, et al. Effect of minimally invasive surfactant therapy vs sham treatment on death or bronchopulmonary dysplasia in preterm infants with respiratory distress syndrome: the OPTIMIST-A randomized clinical trial. *JAMA*. 2021;326(24):2478–87.
12. Abdel-Latif ME, Davis PG, Wheeler KI, et al. Surfactant therapy via thin catheter in preterm infants with or at risk of respiratory distress syndrome. *Cochrane Database Syst Rev*. 2021;(5):CD011672.

Target Ranges of Oxygen Saturation in Extremely Preterm Infants

The SUPPORT Trial

JAMES I. HAGADORN

"A lower target range of oxygenation (85% to 89%), as compared with a higher range (91% to 95%), did not significantly decrease the composite outcome of severe retinopathy or death, but it resulted in an increase in mortality and a substantial decrease in severe retinopathy among survivors."

—CARLO ET AL.[1]

Research Question: Does maintaining a lower (85% to 89%) as compared with higher (91% to 95%) oxygen saturation during routine care reduce the incidence of the composite outcome of severe retinopathy of prematurity or death among infants born between 24 and 27 weeks' gestation?

Why Was This Study Done: For decades, the neonatal community has struggled to balance the risks and benefits of liberal versus restricted oxygen therapy.[2,3] This study was undertaken out of concern that saturations in the higher range of "normal" still posed an increased risk for ROP.

Year Study Began: 2005

Year Study Published: 2010

Study Location: United States (>20 centers within the Neonatal Research Network, NICHD)

Who Was Studied: Infants born between 24 and 27 weeks' gestation for whom a decision had been made to provide full resuscitation.

Who Was Excluded: Infants born at other hospitals and those known to have major congenital anomalies.

How Many Patients: 1316

Study Overview: The SUPPORT (Surfactant, Positive Pressure, and Oxygenation Randomized Trial) trial was part of a worldwide collaboration, a 2-by-2 factorial design, RCT (Figure 16.1). This manuscript reports the results for the comparison of two oxygen saturation target ranges. (Nota bene: The CPAP [continuous positive airway pressure] arm,[4] is discussed in Chapter 15.)

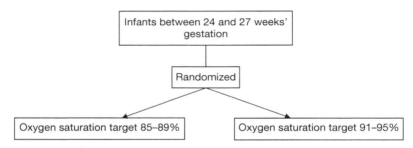

Figure 16.1 Study Overview

Study Interventions: The trial used a 2-by-2 factorial design to randomize infants to 1 of 2 approaches to noninvasive respiratory support initiated in the delivery room, and to 1 of 2 oxygen saturation target ranges during routine NICU care.

- Infants randomized to the lower oxygenation saturation target range received supplemental oxygen titrated to achieve saturations between 85% and 89%.
- Infants randomized to the higher oxygenation saturation target range received supplemental oxygen titrated to achieve saturations between 91% and 95%.

The intervention was started within the first 2 hours after birth and continued until 36 weeks' PMA or until the infant was breathing ambient air and did not require positive pressure support. Blinding was maintained with the use of modified pulse oximeters. Caregivers were instructed to adjust the concentration of oxygen to maintain the displayed values between 88% and 92% in all study participants. Below 85% and above 95% oximeters displayed true values in both groups.

How Long Was Follow-up: Hospital discharge

What Were the Endpoints:
Primary outcomes: Composite outcome of death or severe ROP.
Selected secondary outcomes: BPD, safety outcomes.

Concerns Regarding Bias: The study was at unclear risk for detection/performance bias, as the imperfect design of the study oximeter masking algorithm may have contributed to reduced separation between true saturations in the 2 study groups.[5]

RESULTS

- Infants in the lower oxygen saturation group and those in the higher saturation group did not differ with respect to the primary outcome of severe ROP or death before discharge (adjusted relative risk [aRR] 0.90, 95% CI 0.76 to 1.06, $p = 0.21$).
- Death before discharge occurred in more infants in the lower oxygen saturation group (19.9% versus 16.2%; aRR 1.27, 95% CI 1.01 to 1.60, $p = 0.04$;). This could not be ascribed to an increase in any specific condition. Major causes of death did not differ between the 2 groups.
- The rate of severe ROP among survivors was lower in the lower saturation group (8.6% versus 17.9%; aRR 0.52, 95% CI 0.37 to 0.73, $p <0.001$).
- The duration of mechanical ventilation, CPAP, and nasal synchronized intermittent mandatory ventilation; the rates of BPD among survivors; the composite outcome of BPD or death by 36 weeks did not differ significantly between the treatment groups.

Criticisms and Limitations: Despite sophisticated attempts at blinding, there was less separation of actual saturation values than expected, with a large amount of overlap in saturation ranges between the 2 groups. The median oxygen saturation value in the lower (85%–89%) oxygen saturation was higher than 90%.[1] The precision of oxygen management may have been impacted by multiple factors, including human factors or staffing, as it has been shown in the NICU that higher ratios of patients to nurses can negatively impact the ability to attain oxygen saturation goals.[6] Technical issues, including artifacts in the algorithm used to blind the saturation monitors,[7] may have contributed to the lack of separation. The exact cause or causes of saturation imprecision in this study remain unknown, but the example serves as a reminder of the complex nature of this area of study as well as potential obstacles for incorporating such changes at the NICU level.

Unlike other studies, this trial started within the delivery room. The start of study algorithm from delivery may represent one reason for the unique findings in this study as against those of other oxygen trials.

Other Relevant Studies and Information:
- At follow-up evaluation of this cohort at 18 to 22 months' CA, no significant differences were detected in the composite outcome of death or neurodevelopmental impairment.[8]
- This trial contributed its data to a prospectively planned meta-analysis along with 4 other trials (a collaboration known as NeOProM, the Neonatal Oxygenation Prospective Meta-analysis). The individual participant data from 4965 extremely preterm infants found no difference between the lower and higher SpO_2 targets for the primary composite outcome of death or major disability at 18 to 24 months' CA. Of note, the 4 other studies showed similar effects on death but did not demonstrate a comparable impact on ROP.[9]
- In reviewing these findings, the American Academy of Pediatrics suggested that, at least for some infants, an oxygen saturation target of 90% to 95% appears safer than 85% to 89%.[10]

Summary and Implications: The findings reported by the SUPPORT trial and other NeOProM trials precluded a simple answer regarding a "best" saturation target for supplemental oxygen management in extremely preterm infants. The optimum risk:benefit balance between lower versus higher saturations may vary among NICUs.[11] The ideal saturation target for extremely preterm infants requiring supplemental oxygen therapy remains unclear, but is likely patient-specific, dynamic, and dependent upon a number of patient- and NICU-level variables.

A CONVERSATION WITH THE TRIALIST:
WALDEMAR CARLO

Could you comment on the ethics discussion following publication of this trial, centering on the consent requirements for trials that compare 2 standard therapies for critical illness, in a population for which mortality was not trivial?

There were several discussions on the ethics of the trial including publications in New England Journal of Medicine (NEJM) by the SUPPORT team and the editors of NEJM. There was a National Institutes of Health (NIH) symposium and a conference call with ethicists in the US. There was consensus the trial was well designed and conducted and met ethical concerns.

Here is a sample of the comments by leaders in the field.

- *Benjamin S Wilfond, MD, and over 40 other ethicists and pediatricians published a letter to the editor in NEJM and backed the SUPPORT team, stating: "We urge the Office for Human Research Protections (OHRP) to withdraw its notification to the institutions involved in the Surfactant, Positive Pressure, and Oxygenation Randomized Trial (SUPPORT) that they failed to meet regulatory informed-consent requirements, in particular regarding reasonably foreseeable risks of enrollment in the study. We believe that this conclusion was a substantive error and will have adverse implications for future research."*

- *Kathy Hudson, Alan Guttmacher, and Francis Collins published a letter to the editor in NEJM on behalf of the NIH. Reviewing the prior evidence, they stated: "The more recent studies showed no increased risk of death or neurodevelopmental impairment at saturation levels as low as 70%. Given these data, the investigators had no reason to foresee that infants in one study group would have a higher risk of death than would those in the other group."*

- *Jeffrey Drazen, MD, editor of NEJM and other NEJM editors wrote: "The results of SUPPORT have been critical in informing treatment decisions for extremely preterm infants. When babies like Patrick Bouvier Kennedy are born today, their chances of survival to adulthood are greatly improved, thanks to research made possible by thousands of parents and their children. We are dismayed by the response of the OHRP and consider the SUPPORT trial a model of how to make medical progress."*

References

1. Carlo W, Finer N, Walsh M, et al.; Support Study Group of the Eunice Kennedy Shriver NICHD Neonatal Research Network. Target ranges of oxygen saturation in extremely preterm infants. *N Engl J Med*. 2010;362:1959–69.
2. Duc G, Sinclair JC. Oxygen administration. In: Sinclair JC, Bracken MB, editors. *Effective Care of the Newborn Infant*. Oxford University Press; New York: 1992. pp. 178–94.
3. Bolton DP, Cross KW. Further observations on cost of preventing retrolental fibroplasia. *Lancet*. 1974;303:445–8.
4. Vaucher Y, Peralta-Carcelen M, Finer N, et al.; Support Study Group of the Eunice Kennedy Shriver NICHD Neonatal Research Network. Neurodevelopmental outcomes in the early CPAP and pulse oximetry trial. *N Engl J Med*. 2012;367:2495–504.
5. Schmidt B, Roberts R, Whyte R, et al.; Canadian Oxygen Trial Group. Impact of study oximeter masking algorithm on titration of oxygen therapy in the Canadian Oxygen Trial. *J Pediatr*. 2014;165:666–71 e2.
6. Sink DW, Hope SAE, Hagadorn JI. Nurse:patient ratio and achievement of oxygen saturation goals in premature infants. *Arch Dis Child Fetal Neonatal Ed*. 2011;96:F93–F98.
7. Johnston E, Boyle B, Juszczak E, et al. Oxygen targeting in preterm infants using the masimo set radical pulse oximeter. *Arch Dis Child Fetal Neonatal Ed*. 2011;96:F429–33.
8. Finer N, Carlo W, Walsh M, et al.; Support Study Group of the Eunice Kennedy Shriver NICHD Neonatal Research Network. Early CPAP versus surfactant in extremely preterm infants. *N Engl J Med*. 2010;362:1970–9.
9. Askie L, Darlow B, Finer N, et al.; Neonatal Oxygenation Prospective Meta-analysis Collaboration. Association between oxygen saturation targeting and death or disability in extremely preterm infants in the neonatal oxygenation prospective meta-analysis collaboration. *JAMA*. 2018;319:2190–201.
10. Cummings J, Polin R; American Academy of Pediatrics Committee on Fetus and Newborn. Oxygen targeting in extremely low birth weight infants. *Pediatrics*. 2016;138:e20161576.
11. Schmidt B, Whyte R, Roberts R. Trade-off between lower or higher oxygen saturations for extremely preterm infants: The first Benefits of Oxygen Saturation Targeting (BOOST) II trial reports its primary outcome. *J Pediatr*. 2014;165:6–8.

A Trial Comparing Noninvasive Ventilation Strategies in Preterm Infants

The NIPPV Trial

BRETT J. MANLEY

"Among extremely low-birth-weight infants, the rate of survival to 36 weeks of postmenstrual age without bronchopulmonary dysplasia did not differ significantly after noninvasive respiratory support with nasal intermittent positive pressure ventilation as compared with nasal continuous positive airway pressure."

—KIRPALANI ET AL.[1]

Research Question: In extremely low birth weight (ELBW, <1000 grams) infants, does using nasal intermittent positive pressure ventilation (NIPPV) for respiratory support, compared with nasal continuous positive airway pressure (nCPAP), improve the rate of survival without BPD at 36 weeks' PMA?

Why Was This Study Done: NIPPV and nCPAP are the 2 most commonly used forms of noninvasive respiratory support. However, prior to this trial, comparisons between the 2 were limited to small trials with inconsistent results for preventing BPD.

Year Study Began: 2007

Year Study Published: 2013

Study Location: Canada, Qatar, United Kingdom, United States of America, Sweden, Singapore, Republic of Ireland, The Netherlands, Belgium, and Austria. (34 centers total)

Who Was Studied: ELBW infants born < 30 weeks' gestation who were candidates for noninvasive respiratory support, either as initial support between birth and 7 days of life or after the initial extubation from mechanical support during the first 28 days of life.

Who Was Excluded: Infants who were expected to die, had congenital abnormalities (including any airway abnormality), required surgery, or had a neuromuscular disorder.

How Many Patients: 1009

Study Overview: The NIPPV Trial was a parallel-group, unmasked RCT (Figure 17.1).

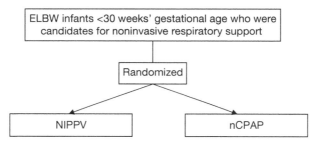

Figure 17.1 Study Overview

What Were the Interventions:
- Infants randomized to NIPPV received respiratory support via any technique that combined nCPAP with an intermittent increase in applied pressure. Synchronization of NIPPV "inflations" with the infant's breathing was permitted but not mandated. Infants randomized to nCPAP received this form of respiratory support without intermittent increases in applied pressure allowed.
- Infants whose condition could not be maintained with the assigned method of noninvasive respiratory support were reintubated, and the originally assigned intervention was resumed after extubation. Guidelines for initial and maximal settings, and for weaning of

respiratory support were provided to the study sites, although clinicians could individualize care.

How Long Was Follow-up: Hospital discharge

What Were the Endpoints:
Primary outcome: Composite outcome of death or BPD at 36 weeks' PMA.
Selected secondary outcomes: Reintubation, PMA at extubation, PMA at weaning from any respiratory support, air leak, brain injury, retinopathy of prematurity, nasal trauma.

Concerns Regarding Bias: The study was at high risk for performance/detection bias, as caregivers were not blinded to the intervention. However, the outcome of BPD was assessed independently via oxygen reduction test.

RESULTS
- There was no difference in the primary outcome of death or BPD (NIPPV 38.4% versus nCPAP 36.7%; adjusted odds ratio 1.09, 95% CI 0.83 to 1.43, $p = 0.56$).
- There were no differences in the individual components of the primary outcome, or in the frequencies of other secondary outcomes, including potential adverse effects of treatment.
- Post-randomization intubation was required for 58.3% of surviving infants in the NIPPV group and 59.1% in the nCPAP group.
- In preplanned subgroup analyses there were no significant interactions between treatment assignment and center, birth weight, or prior-intubation status.

Criticisms and Limitations: It was not feasible to blind the intervention, leaving a potential for bias, especially as clinicians had discretion in how they managed the respiratory support (although there were clinical guidelines for weaning, extubation, and reintubation). Ultimately, the rate of adherence to the assigned treatment was high, but there was some crossover between groups: infants in the NIPPV group received a median 6 days of nCPAP, and almost 10% of the nCPAP group received some NIPPV. This may have obscured any difference in effectiveness between the 2 therapies.

Whilst the NIPPV Trial is the largest trial evaluating the use of NIPPV as respiratory support for ELBW/very preterm infants, it perhaps raises as many questions as it answers due to its heterogeneous entry criteria and interventions. The pathophysiology present in infants treated for primary lung disease differs substantially from that of those managed post-extubation. Evidence of differential effectiveness of NIPPV dependent on the peak inspiratory pressures used and on the use of synchronization was evident in previous trials and meta-analyses. It is possible that the NIPPV Trial failed to detect real differences between the 2 most commonly used forms of noninvasive support.

Other Relevant Studies and Information:

- The NIPPV Trial differs from smaller studies in that it recruited a heterogeneous study population and permitted a variety of devices to deliver NIPPV, including some that delivered synchronized "inflations" with the infant's spontaneous breaths.
- The NIPPV Cochrane Reviews (also co-authored by Kirpalani) have shown that, compared with all other noninvasive approaches, NIPPV significantly lowers the risk for intubation and mechanical ventilation in preterm infants, when pooled with many other smaller trials; this effect is found when NIPPV is used either as primary therapy for respiratory distress syndrome or as post-extubation support.[2,3] However, these findings did not translate into reductions in more important outcomes such as death or BPD. [2,3]
- When analyzed by synchronization with the infant's spontaneous breathing (synchronized NIPPV versus unsynchronized), a benefit from synchronization is <u>not</u> consistently found when used as primary therapy of respiratory distress syndrome.[2] However, there appears to be a strong signal favoring synchronized NIPPV in reducing extubation failure when used for post-extubation support of preterm infants, both in the Cochrane Review[3] and in a network meta-analysis by Ramaswamy et al.[4]
- A promising approach to synchronization of NIPPV is neurally adjusted ventilatory assist (NAVA), that synchronizes respiratory support via the electrical activity of the diaphragm. Several small RCTs comparing NAVA-NIPPV with nCPAP have been reported.[5-7] Though the results are mixed, these studies indicate that larger trials evaluating this technique are warranted.

Summary and Implications: The NIPPV Trial did not find a benefit of using NIPPV as respiratory support for ELBW/very preterm infants. This large, pragmatic trial allowed the use of both synchronized and non-synchronized NIPPV.

Evidence from other studies suggests a benefit of using synchronized NIPPV, and further large trials are required to guide clinicians as to the optimal mode of noninvasive support for very preterm infants.

A CONVERSATION WITH THE TRIALIST: HARESH KIRPALANI

What are the pros and cons of conducting such a pragmatic study?

The major advantage is a proximity to the real world of clinical bedside practice. With fewer restrictions and rules, the results apply better to the setting of the "standard" clinician. Perhaps the major disadvantage of the pragmatic study is its inability to study precise mechanisms. For example, we allowed the use of synchronized as well as non-synchronized devices, but did not have sufficient statistical power to study the treatment effects conclusively in those subgroups. This introduces the potential aid from larger trials—enabling a priori *subgroup analysis to overcome some of this problem. However, at the time we did the NIPPV study, we were aiming to address whether a simple, cheap, and available potential means of applying non-synchronized NIPPV would be of help. In addition, at the time good, approved synchronizers were not available.*

What are the most important questions about NIPPV to be teased out in the next clinical trials?

Whether or not synchronization helps both time to extubation, but also whether it reduces rates of BPD. There are ancillary queries about mode of fixation of devices, and potential for nasal trauma. However, the latter is very likely most influenced by nursing care ratios. If the essential question of a benefit of a mode of synchronization is indeed shown, then would come the next question: query of method of synchronization. At the moment, the main contenders are flow-based triggering and diaphragmatic based triggering.

References

1. Kirpalani H, Millar D, Lemyre B, et al. A trial comparing noninvasive ventilation strategies in preterm infants. *N Engl J Med.* 2013;369(7):611–20.
2. Lemyre B, Laughon M, Bose C, et al. Early nasal intermittent positive pressure ventilation (NIPPV) versus early nasal continuous positive airway pressure (NCPAP) for preterm infants. *Cochrane Database Syst Rev.* 2016;12:CD005384.
3. Lemyre B, Davis PG, De Paoli AG, et al. Nasal intermittent positive pressure ventilation (NIPPV) versus nasal continuous positive airway pressure (NCPAP) for preterm neonates after extubation. *Cochrane Database Syst Rev.* 2017;2:CD003212.

4. Ramaswamy VV, More K, Roehr CC, et al. Efficacy of noninvasive respiratory support modes for primary respiratory support in preterm neonates with respiratory distress syndrome: Systematic review and network meta-analysis. *Pediatr Pulmonol.* 2020;55(11):2940–63.
5. Kallio M, Mahlman M, Koskela U, et al. NIV NAVA versus nasal CPAP in premature infants: a randomized clinical trial. *Neonatology.* 2019;116(4):380–4.
6. Yagui AC, Meneses J, Zólio BA, et al. Nasal continuous positive airway pressure (NCPAP) or noninvasive neurally adjusted ventilatory assist (NIV-NAVA) for preterm infants with respiratory distress after birth: a randomized controlled trial. *Pediatr Pulmonol.* 2019;54(11):1704–11.
7. Makker K, Cortez J, Jha K, et al. Comparison of extubation success using noninvasive positive pressure ventilation (NIPPV) versus noninvasive neurally adjusted ventilatory assist (NI-NAVA). *J Perinatol.* 2020;40(8):1202–10.

High-Flow Nasal Cannulae in Very Preterm Infants After Extubation

The HIPERSPACE Trial

CHARLES CHRISTOPH ROEHR

". . . it seems reasonable to use high-flow nasal cannulae initially after extubation if both therapies [high-flow nasal cannulae and nasal CPAP] are available."

—MANLEY ET AL.[1]

Research Question: For very preterm infants receiving noninvasive respiratory support following extubation from mechanical ventilation, is high-flow nasal cannula (HFNC) an appropriate alternative to nasal continuous positive airway pressure (CPAP), to prevent re-intubation?

Why Was This Study Done: At the time of this study, there was the beginning of a practice-change towards using HFNC to prevent respiratory failure following extubation, for which trial evidence was lacking.

Year Study Began: 2010

Year Study Published: 2013

Study Location: Australia (3 centers)

Who Was Studied: Very premature infants <32 weeks' gestation, receiving mechanical ventilation and considered ready for extubation.

Who Was Excluded: Infants with PMA >36 weeks at the time of extubation, infants with major congenital anomalies, or infants for whom maximal intensive care was not being provided.

How Many Patients: 303. A sample size of 300 infants was calculated to show a 20% margin of non-inferiority of HFNC treatment with a power of 87%.

Study Overview: The HIPERSPACE trial was an unmasked, non-inferiority RCT (Figure 18.1). Stratification was by gestational age (GA) group (<26 weeks' versus ≥26 weeks' GA) and by study center.

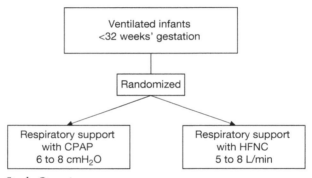

Figure 18.1 Study Overview

What Were the Interventions:
- Infants randomized to CPAP received nasal CPAP at a pressure range of 6 to 8 cm H_2O following extubation. In this group, non-synchronized nasal intermittent positive pressure ventilation (NIPPV) could be used at any time.
- Infants randomized to HFNC received HFNC at 5 to 8 L/min following extubation.

Weaning from respiratory support was permitted once clinically stable >24 hours on minimal settings (HFNC <2 L/min or CPAP <5 cm H_2O) and fraction of inspired oxygen (FiO2) <0.3.

Respiratory support could be escalated if clinically indicated, from HFNC to CPAP/NIPPV to re-intubation.

How Long Was Follow-up: Hospital discharge

What Were the Endpoints:
Primary outcome: Intubation within 7 days.
Selected secondary outcomes: Death, pneumothorax, duration of respiratory support, length of hospital stay.

Concerns Regarding Bias: The trial was at high risk for performance/detection bias, as caregivers were not blinded to the intervention. This is especially relevant as the decision to escalate or de-escalate treatment included physician's discretion.

RESULTS

- On average, infants in both groups were extubated after 36 hours of ventilation.
- HFNC was deemed noninferior to CPAP for post-extubation respiratory support, with infants supported with HFNC experiencing a failure rate of 34.2% compared with 25.8% in the CPAP group (risk difference [RD] 8.4%; 95% CI −1.9 to 18.7).
- Infants most often failed due to persistent apnea, irrespective of allocation treatment.
- In infants with GA <26 weeks' GA ($n = 62$), failure rate was high in both treatment groups, but the RD was 20% in favor of CPAP (95% CI −1.9 to 41.8).
- Apart from less nasal trauma in the HFNC group, no statistically significant difference was observed between groups for secondary outcomes.

Criticisms and Limitations: This is one of the very first non-inferiority trials in the neonatal literature.[2] Although, at the time of the trial, CPAP and, increasingly, HFNC were being used to facilitate extubation, the physical properties of HFNC would not suggest superiority.[3,4] Considering potential disadvantages of CPAP therapy, including increased rates of nasal skin erosion and necrosis,[5] even a marginal but tolerable inferiority in efficacy might provide a sufficiently convincing argument to establish HFNC as an alternative to CPAP. Using a non-inferiority design allows the investigation of whether the new intervention offers marginal advantages in one aspect of care. Often these new interventions present other important advantages to the current standard treatment, such as improved safety, convenience, better compliance, or cost.[6] Conversely, a disadvantage of non-inferiority trial design in this study is that the non-inferiority margin (NIM) was, by the authors' own account, somewhat arbitrarily defined. Overall, an 8.4% absolute risk difference for extubation failure may convince many parents and caregivers who prefer a less injurious form of noninvasive respiratory support for their babies and are willing to consider that in some babies, treatment may have to be escalated to CPAP. Others may not feel convinced that this result mandates a practice change.

The trial was under-powered to show non-inferiority in the most premature infants, those <26 weeks' GA. For these patients, who are the most frequently ventilated patient group, there is still a dearth of evidence to define the most appropriate form of respiratory support.[7] Appropriately, Manley and co-authors caution on the use of HFNC as the first-line respiratory support after extubation in the most premature babies.

Other Relevant Studies and Information:
- The most recent Cochrane review,[8] which includes 15 studies and represents >1700 infants, compared CPAP to HFNC for post-extubation respiratory support and concluded comparable efficacy of both treatments for important outcomes, including treatment failure, re-intubation rate, BPD, and death. Further, pneumothorax rate and nasal trauma were significantly less prevalent in infants supported by HFNC, compared with CPAP.
- Currently, HFNC is considered a valid alternative to CPAP for preventing re-intubation for most preterm infants.[9]
- However, trials from the same group of investigators have addressed the question of HFNC versus CPAP for primary respiratory support.[10] The HIPSTER trial, another non-inferiority trial investigating initial CPAP versus HFNC in preterm infants, found HFNC inferior to CPAP, with the pre-specified non-inferiority margin of 10% for treatment failure.

Summary and Implications: This innovative trial in neonatology demonstrated HFNC to be noninferior to CPAP as post-extubation support, validating HFNC as an alternative to CPAP for preventing re-intubation. Many embraced HFNC for its ease of use and increased patient comfort. However, further evidence is needed for the use of HFNC in the most premature infants.

A CONVERSATION WITH THE TRIALIST: BRETT J. MANLEY

Could you walk us through some of your team's considerations in determining what constitutes non-inferiority?

We decided to perform a non-inferiority trial as clinicians were already opting to use HFNC due to its perceived advantages of ease-of-use, less nasal trauma, and improved infant tolerance. We pre-specified the margin of non-inferiority for HFNC as a fairly generous 20 percentage points above the treatment failure rate for nasal CPAP . . . .

Whilst the choice of 20% was rather arbitrary, and feasibility was a consideration, our consensus was that if 20% more infants reached treatment failure criteria during HFNC, but suffered less nasal trauma, were more comfortable, were potentially "rescued" from re-intubation by subsequent nasal CPAP (ultimately this occurred approximately half the time), and meanwhile did not suffer a major clinical deterioration or acidosis (ultimately 95% of the HFNC group vs 96% of the nasal CPAP group did not), then HFNC might be an acceptable alternative therapy.

*This trial does not offer conclusive evidence **in favor** of the use of HFNC over nasal CPAP. It does, however, suggest that HFNC is a viable alternative to nasal CPAP, at least in the more mature subgroup of very preterm infants, that does not cause harm and may offer novel advantages. Ultimately, each clinician will appraise the results and make a decision whether to apply (or, in some cases, **continue** to apply) HFNC for preterm infants as post-extubation support.*

The trade-offs of nursing and parent preferences for ease of handling the infant are interesting considerations in comparing these 2 methods of respiratory support; in your clinical practice, how do you balance these interests with the available comparative evidence?

In our current clinical practice we extubate all extremely preterm infants to CPAP, and more mature infants to HFNC. For extremely preterm infants extubated to CPAP, we subsequently aim to change them to HFNC 6–7 L/min when they are receiving CPAP 6 cm H_2O or less and with supplemental oxygen requirements <30%—and we note the parents' and nurses' satisfaction when we do so!

References

1. Manley BJ, Owen LS, Doyle LW, et al. High-flow nasal cannulae in very preterm infants after extubation. *N Engl J Med*. 2013;369:1425–33.
2. Piaggio G, Elbourne DR, Altman DG, et al.; CONSORT Group. Reporting of noninferiority and equivalence randomized trials: an extension of the CONSORT statement. *JAMA*. 2006;295:1152–60.
3. Wilkinson DJ, Andersen CC, Smith K, et al. Pharyngeal pressure with high-flow nasal cannulae in premature infants. *J Perinatol*. 2008;28:42–7.
4. Lavizzari A, Veneroni C, Colnaghi M, et al. Respiratory mechanics during NCPAP and HHHFNC at equal distending pressures. *Arch Dis Child Fetal Neonatal Ed*. 2014;99:F315–20.

5. Mahmoud RA, Schmalisch G, Oswal A, et al. Non-invasive ventilatory support in neonates: an evidence-based update. *Paediatr Respir Rev.* 2022;44:11–18.
6. Hahn S. Understanding noninferiority trials. *Korean J Pediatr.* 2012;55:403–7.
7. Wright CJ, Glaser K, Speer CP, et al. Noninvasive ventilation and exogenous surfactant in times of ever decreasing gestational age: how do we make the most of these tools? *J Pediatr.* 2022;247:138–46.
8. Wilkinson D, Andersen C, O'Donnell CPF, et al. High flow nasal cannula for respiratory support in preterm infants. *Cochrane Database Syst Rev.* 2016;(2):CD006405.
9. Dani C. Nasal continuous positive airway pressure and high-flow nasal cannula today. *Clin Perinatol.* 2021;48:711–24.
10. Roberts CT, Owen LS, Manley BJ, et al.; HIPSTER Trial Investigators. Nasal high-flow therapy for primary respiratory support in preterm infants. *N Engl J Med.* 2016;375:1142–51.

Nutrition

19

Randomized Trial of Early Diet in Preterm Babies and Later Intelligence Quotient

MICHELLE FERNANDES AND JON DORLING

"We have designed a series of randomised prospective studies to test the vulnerability of the brain to suboptimal nutrition during specific periods of [the critical spurt in brain growth]."

—LUCAS ET AL.[1]

Research Question: Does the type of formula (standard versus preterm) fed to preterm infants during the first 4 weeks of life, either as their sole diet or as a supplement to maternal breast milk, influence intelligence quotient (IQ) scores during mid-childhood?

Why Was This Study Done: The early brain critical spurt in preterm infants could be affected by early feeding composition. This study was among a series of publications by the same research group to evaluate the causal effects of early nutrition on long-term neurodevelopment of preterm infants.[2,3]

Year Study Began: 1982

Year Study Published: 1998

Study Location: United Kingdom (2 centers total)

Who Was Studied: Infants born preterm, who weighed <1850g at birth.

Who Was Excluded: Infants with major congenital malformations known to impair growth or development.

How Many Patients: 424, of whom 377 survived. A total of 355 were fully assessed at 7.5 to 8 years.

Study Overview: This study was a parallel-group RCT (Figure 19.1), with randomization stratified by maternal preference for breast milk (Trial A, Trial B) and then further stratified by birth weight (<1200g, ≥1200g).[2]

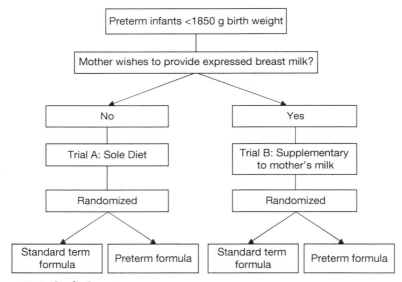

Figure 19.1 Study Overview

What Were the Interventions:
- Trial A—Infants whose mothers chose not to provide breast milk were randomized to receive either a standard term formula or a preterm formula "designed" to meet the increased nutritional needs of preterm infants. This design gave more protein and fat with a resulting higher caloric intake (0.334 versus 0.284 MJ/100 mL).
- Trial B—Infants whose mothers chose to provide breast milk were randomized to receive either the standard term or the preterm formula, as a supplement to maternal breast milk.

Trial diets were discontinued at hospital discharge or when body weights of 2000 g were achieved, whichever was sooner. The median study duration was approximately 4 weeks.

How Long Was Follow-up: 7.5 to 8 years

What Were the Endpoints:
Primary outcome: Overall IQ measured on the Wechsler intelligence scale for children (revised).
Secondary outcomes: Separate components of IQ scores; children with a severe developmental outcome, defined as the prevalence of cerebral palsy (CP) or verbal IQ score <85.

Concerns Regarding Bias: The study was at considerable risk of bias in the context of multiple secondary analyses with insufficient power. Additionally, the reporting appears biased, largely basing conclusions on subgroups. Finally, the authors appropriately declare manufacturers' funding.

RESULTS

- There was no difference in the primary outcome of overall IQ scores at 7.5 to 8 years between children who had received preterm formula versus standard either as their sole diet (2.2 point advantage; 95% CI −2.7 to 7.0) or as a supplement to mother's milk (1.0; 95% CI −3.0 to 5.0).
- With regard to secondary outcomes, verbal IQ scores were similar between groups.
- Subgroup analyses suggested benefit for male infants, especially those who received the highest intakes of the trial diet, with the most benefit observed in verbal IQ scores.

Criticisms and Limitations: The authors of this trial rely heavily on subgroup analyses to bolster the impact of early dietary manipulation on later cognitive function, emphasizing in their reporting the effect seen on boys and those with the highest intake of trial diets. This interpretation is risky. As smaller subsets of randomized groups, subgroups are more prone to bias from subtle imbalances. Additionally, the risk of a false positive result is increased as more comparisons are added to a study. A recent analysis revealed that reproduction of results found by subgroup analysis was unlikely.[4]

Perhaps these shortcomings were not appreciated at the time, since the reported findings of this trial led to rapid changes in NICU practice, with enriched formula becoming standard of care. The lesser touted and more meaningful impact of this trial was in its innovative approach of studying the effects of nutritional interventions on childhood development after preterm birth. It revolutionized the community's approach to preterm nutrition. Importantly these authors achieved an impressive follow-up at 7.5 to 8 years of 98% survivors still in the UK, likely because of the unified health care system in the UK at that time.

Other Relevant Studies and Information:
- The authors' initial publication of 18-month outcomes of this cohort demonstrated improved developmental testing in infants assigned to preterm formula, and formed the basis of this study. It also relied on subgroup analysis suggesting a greater effect in male infants.[2]
- A recent study evaluating preterm versus standard formula in the post-discharge period showed no impact on cognition at 10-year follow-up.[5]
- In this trial cohort, another secondary analysis reported higher IQ in children whose early diet included their own mother's milk (trial B) compared with those fed solely on formula (trial A).[3] However, overall evidence on the developmental impact of breast milk versus formula for preterm infants remains scarce.[6]
- There have been no other trials evaluating the impact of early preterm formula versus standard formula on childhood neurodevelopmental outcomes. The most recent Cochrane review on the topic expresses uncertainty that clinicians and families would support further study on the topic, as early nutrient-enriched formula is now widely established.[7]

Summary and Implications: This trial was groundbreaking in its effort to study the long-term neurodevelopmental effects of dietary manipulations for preterm infants. However serious validity issues are raised. Despite questionable interpretation, the trial reframed the neonatal community's perception of early diet and potential for long-term effects, leading the way for further dietary studies powered for neurodevelopmental outcomes.

A FEW WORDS FROM THE EDITOR

There are arguably few studies that have influenced practice more than Lucas and colleagues' study on the effects of early nutrition on long-term neurodevelopment of preterm infants. Although the intervention led to no difference in the primary outcome of overall IQ scores at 7.5 to 8 years, many have embraced the notion that early nutrition strongly influences intellectual development based on certain subgroup analyses. While these findings should be viewed with a degree of uncertainty, for many, they told us what we wanted to hear.

—Roger Soll

References

1. Lucas A, Morley R, Cole TJ. Randomised trial of early diet in preterm babies and later intelligence quotient. *BMJ.* 1998 Nov 28;317(7171):1481–7.
2. Lucas A, Morley R, Cole TJ, et al. Early diet in preterm babies and developmental status at 18 months. *Lancet.* 1990;335:1477–81.
3. Lucas A, Morley R, Cole TJ, et al. Breast milk and subsequent intelligence quotient in children born preterm. *Lancet.* 1992;339(8788):261–4.
4. Wallach JD, Sullivan PG, Trepanowski JF. Evaluation of evidence of statistical support and corroboration of subgroup claims in randomized clinical trials. *JAMA Intern Med.* 2017;177(4):554–60.
5. Embleton ND, Wood CL, Pearce MS, et al. Early diet in preterm infants and later cognition: 10-year follow-up of a randomized controlled trial. *Pediatr Res.* 2021;89:1442–6.
6. Brown JV, Walsh V, McGuire W. Formula versus maternal breast milk for feeding preterm or low birth weight infants. *Cochrane Database Syst Rev.* 2019;(8):CD002972.
7. Walsh V, Brown JVE, Askie LM, et al. Nutrient-enriched formula versus standard formula for preterm infants. *Cochrane Database Syst Rev.* 2019;(7):CD004204.

20

Vitamin A Supplementation for Extremely Low Birth Weight Infants

AXEL R. FRANZ AND SUSANNE HAY

"Our findings support the use of [vitamin A supplementation] for extremely low-birth-weight infants who require early respiratory support."
—Tyson et al.[1]

Research Question: Does vitamin A supplementation, compared with placebo, in extremely low-birth-weight (ELBW) infants increase the rate of survival without BPD at 36 weeks' PMA, without causing harm?

Why Was This Study Done: Extremely preterm infants are at risk for deficiency of vitamin A.[2] The pathological changes of BPD are similar to those observed in vitamin A–deficient experimental animals.

Year Study Began: 1996

Year Study Published: 1999

Study Location: United States (14 centers)

Who Was Studied: Infants with birth weights between 401 g and 1000 g who received mechanical ventilation or supplemental oxygen at 24 hours of life.

Who Was Excluded: Infants with major congenital anomalies or congenital nonbacterial infections, and those considered nonviable or who were to receive vitamin A in a parenteral fat emulsion or in doses exceeding recommendations for multivitamin preparations.

How Many Patients: 807

Study Overview: This was a parallel-group, randomized RCT (Figure 20.1).

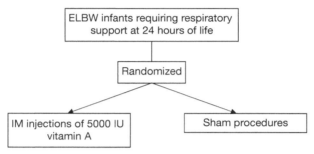

Figure 20.1 Study Overview

What Were the Interventions:
- Infants in the vitamin A group received 5000 IU (1500 µg) vitamin A intramuscularly (IM) 3 times per week for 4 weeks.
- Infants in the control group received sham procedures (without injections).

How Long Was Follow-up: 36 weeks' PMA, 18 to 22 months' CA.

What Were the Endpoints:
Primary outcome: Composite outcome of death or BPD (defined as need for supplemental oxygen at 36 weeks' PMA) by 36 weeks' PMA.
Selected secondary outcomes: Sepsis, vitamin A deficiency.

Concerns Regarding Bias: The study was overall at low risk of bias due to effective blinding of the intervention.

RESULTS

- The primary outcome—death or BPD at 36 weeks' PMA—occurred in fewer infants in the vitamin A group than in the control group (55% versus 62%; adjusted RR 0.89, 95% CI 0.80 to 0.99, *p* = 0.03). The reduction in the rate of the composite primary outcome was mostly due to a reduced rate of BPD in survivors (47% versus 56%; RR 0.85, 95% CI 0.73 to 0.98, $p = 0.03$).

- The proportion of infants with serum retinol values below 20 μg/dL (0.70 μmol/L), indicating suboptimal levels, at 28 days was lower in the vitamin A group than in the control group (25% versus 54%, p <0.001).

- There was no clinical or biochemical evidence of vitamin A toxicity. The proportions of infants in the vitamin A group and the control group who had signs of potential vitamin A toxicity were similar.

Criticisms and Limitations: In the 25 years since the start of this trial, respiratory and nutritional management of ELBW infants has changed considerably, with many of these infants now managed on noninvasive respiratory support. It is unclear how these changes in respiratory support might have impacted the results of this trial. Additionally, generalizability concerns have been raised with later cumulative evidence suggesting that the benefit of vitamin A supplementation is limited to infants with baseline low vitamin A intake (See Other Relevant Studies and Information.). Moreover the "fortuitous" experiment of withdrawal of vitamin A from the US markets was not associated with a rise in BPD rates.[3]

Despite parenteral vitamin A supplementation, considerable numbers of infants still had borderline plasma retinol concentrations and biochemical evidence of low hepatic stores. Although increasing liver vitamin A stores, intramuscular vitamin A supplementation did not significantly increase pulmonary stores of vitamin A in a small group of ELBW infants studied post mortem. Hence, the vitamin A dose in the intervention group may still have been too low.

Other Relevant Studies and Information:
- At 18 to 22 months' CA, the primary follow-up outcome of survival without neurodevelopmental impairment did not differ between the comparison groups.[4]
- A recent systematic review supported a beneficial effect of vitamin A for decreasing BPD at 36 weeks' PMA. However, subgroup analysis suggested this may be limited to infants with baseline vitamin A intake <1500 IU/kg/d. Additionally, enteral supplementation may be equally effective as parenteral supplementation.[5]
- Despite evidence of benefit, early vitamin A supplementation of extremely preterm infants has not been widely adopted into common practice.[6] Repeated intramuscular administration are painful and could theoretically increase the risk of infections. The justification of 12 injections to every ELBW infant for modest improvement in short-term

respiratory outcome (and without evidence of longer-term respiratory benefit at 18–22 months) has been questioned.[2]
- Contrary to expectations, a recent reanalysis of this trial indicated that vitamin A supplementation had the greatest benefit for infants who were at the lowest risk of BPD.[7] However, this idiosyncratic post hoc finding should be interpreted with caution.[8]
- A RCT of enteral vitamin A (5000 IU/kg/d) during the first 4 weeks after birth in Germany and Austria completed recruitment to target sample size of 915 ELBW infants in January 2022.[9]

Summary and Implications: This trial provided evidence for vitamin A supplementation as one of the few therapies effective in preventing BPD. However, this approach to vitamin A supplementation has not been universally incorporated into clinical practice. Despite reports of efficacy, the frequency and invasiveness of the tested approach may not achieve what families and caregivers consider the minimally important difference.

A CONVERSATION WITH THE TRIALIST: JON E. TYSON

Having contributed one of very few studies that showed significant reduction in BPD, what is your reaction to the low clinical uptake of this regimen? What are the issues that have prevented uptake of vitamin A in at-risk infants?

The perception that supplemental vitamin A has had little benefit was presumably due partly to an editor of the New England Journal of Medicine inserting the word slightly into the conclusion of the trial abstract: "Vitamin A supplementation slightly [italics mine] decreased the risk of chronic lung disease." (This insertion occurred without the knowledge or agreement of the authors after the galley proofs had been returned.) Yet, a NNT [number needed to treat] of 14 to benefit one patient is considerably smaller than the NNT for many widely recommended therapies used throughout medical practice.

Factors that impede or facilitate the implementation of effective therapies have not been well studied, and implementation science is an important developing area of research. However, the uptake of vitamin A supplementation has been reduced by the scarcity of injectable vitamin A between 2010 and 2014, the large increase in its price over time, and the concern about potential adverse effects from the pain with IM injections of vitamin A (3 times per week for 4 weeks in the Network trial). Pain has been a neglected issue in neonatal trials, and a limitation of the trial was that we made no effort to assess infant distress or at least tabulate the number of painful procedures in a sample of infants. However, with less BPD and a somewhat lower proportion of infants who received antibiotics for >5 days (38% vs. 42%), the vitamin A group could well have experienced similar or even less distress from respiratory disease, infections, or hypoxemic episodes and/or fewer painful procedures from skin punctures for blood gas determinations, CBCs, blood cultures, antibiotics, or IVs.

Do you see opportunities to more individualized vitamin A supplementation for the future?

Who should receive vitamin A supplementation is certainly open to question. Contrary to expectation, a recent post hoc reanalysis of the Network trial found that the effect of supplementation was greater in lower risk than higher risk infants (Rysavy 2021).[7] Routine assessment of vitamin A status may not be very helpful as the effect of factors other than vitamin A deficiency may obscure, modify, or prevent respiratory benefits from vitamin A supplementation. It could be that ELBW infants who don't require respiratory support at 24 hours or infants whose birth weight is, say 1000–1500 g (and wouldn't have been eligible for the Network trial) might have the greatest or most obvious benefit despite their relatively favorable A status at birth. Tools to estimate the likelihood of benefit will require multiple variables assessed in larger, more recent trials.

With the myriad of changes in perinatal care and the smaller and more immature infants treated in NICUs, further research is clearly needed to assess effects of different regimens on lung function, ROP, rates of infection, neurodevelopmental outcome. Recent evidence suggests that enteral vitamin A can be equally if not more effective than IM vitamin A supplementation in reducing BPD and would avoid concerns about pain from injections. However, the appropriate dosing regimen is unclear.

References

1. Tyson JE, Wright LL, Oh W, et al. Vitamin A supplementation for extremely-low-birth-weight infants. National Institute of Child Health and Human Development Neonatal Research Network. *N Engl J Med.* 1999;340(25):1962–8.
2. Mactier H, Weaver LT. Vitamin A and preterm infants: what we know, what we don't know, and what we need to know. *Arch Dis Child Fetal Neonatal Ed.* 2005;90(2):F103–8.
3. Tolia VN, Murthy K, McKinley PS, et al. The effect of the national shortage of vitamin A on death or chronic lung disease in extremely low-birth-weight infants. *JAMA Pediatr.* 2014;168(11):1039–1044.
4. Ambalavanan N, Tyson JE, Kennedy KA, et al. Vitamin A supplementation for extremely low birth weight infants: outcome at 18 to 22 months. *Pediatrics.* 2005;115(3):e249–54.
5. Rakshasbhuvankar AA, Pillow JJ, Simmer KN, et al. Vitamin A supplementation in very-preterm or very-low-birth-weight infants to prevent morbidity and

mortality: a systematic review and meta-analysis of randomized trials. *Am J Clin Nutr.* 2021;114(6):2084–96.

6. Ambalavanan N, Kennedy K, Tyson J, et al. Survey of vitamin A supplementation for extremely-low-birth-weight infants: is clinical practice consistent with the evidence? J Pediatr. 2004;145(3):304–7.

7. Rysavy MA, Li L, Tyson JE, et al. Should vitamin A injections to prevent bronchopulmonary dysplasia or death be reserved for high-risk infants? Reanalysis of the National Institute of Child Health and Human Development Neonatal Research Network Randomized Trial. *J Pediatr.* 2021;236:78–85 e5.

8. Schandelmaier S, Briel M, Varadhan R, et al. Development of the Instrument to assess the Credibility of Effect Modification Analyses (ICEMAN) in randomized controlled trials and meta-analyses. *CMAJ.* 2020;192(32):E901–E906.

9. Meyer S, Kronfeld K, Graber S, et al. Vitamin A to prevent bronchopulmonary dysplasia: the NeoVitaA trial. *J Matern Fetal Neonatal Med.* 2013;26(5):544–5.

21

Promotion of Breastfeeding Intervention Trial. A Randomized Trial in the Republic of Belarus

The PROBIT Trial

NICHOLAS D. EMBLETON

"PROBIT provides an essential scientific underpinning, not only for the Baby-Friendly Hospital Initiative [BFHI], but for future breastfeeding promotion interventions in both developed and developing country settings."

—KRAMER ET AL.[1]

Research Question: Can breastfeeding promotion improve breastfeeding duration and exclusivity and also reduce gastrointestinal and respiratory infection and atopic eczema among infants?

Why Was This Study Done: Prior to this trial, there were no similar studies of this size and nature on breastfeeding. Recommendations for breastfeeding were based on the benefits reported by observational studies.

Year Study Began: 1996

Year Study Published: 2001

Study Location: Republic of Belarus (31 centers)

Who Was Studied: Healthy, singleton, full-term infants weighing ≥2500 g at birth, and their mothers

Who Was Excluded: Mothers for whom breastfeeding was undesirable or contraindicated; infants with Apgar scores <5 at 5 minutes.

How Many Patients: 17,046 mother–infant pairs were enrolled at 31 maternal hospitals and their associated clinics. Of these mother–infant pairs, 16,492 (96.7%) were assessed at 12 months (m).

Study Overview: PROBIT (Promotion of Breastfeeding Intervention Trial) was a cluster-randomized controlled trial (Figure 21.1).

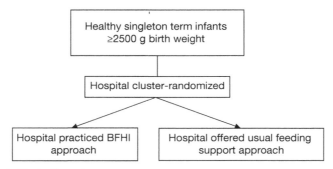

Figure 21.1 Study Overview

What Were the Interventions:
- Hospitals randomized to the intervention arm implemented the Baby-Friendly Hospital Initiative (BFHI) approach. BFHI was developed by the World Health Organization (WHO) and United Nations Children's Fund (UNICEF) as "Ten Steps to Successful Breastfeeding." BFHI emphasizes healthcare worker assistance with initiating and maintaining breastfeeding and lactation and postnatal breastfeeding support.[2]
- Control hospitals continued standard infant feeding practices and policies as used in Belarus at the time of the study.

How Long Was Follow-up: 12 m

What Were the Endpoints:
Primary outcome: Breastfeeding prevalence, as indicated by 3 months of any breastfeeding. However, the added outcome of GI infection was adopted, for which the authors performed a priori sample size estimates.

Selected secondary outcomes: Two or more episodes of any respiratory tract infection; atopic eczema; recurrent wheezing; other measures of breastfeeding duration and exclusivity.

Concerns Regarding Bias: This study was at unclear risk for performance/ascertainment bias. Data was collected by clinical staff who were also responsible for delivering the intervention; however, their adherence and accuracy was determined by an audit involving chart review and maternal interview. There was additional risk for other bias, as it is uncertain whether practices in control sites may have changed during the study if they became aware of practices in intervention sites (spillover effect). However, this would be expected to lessen differences between the groups and unlikely therefore to change conclusions. Fraud was detected in one site by alert monitoring, and that site data was excluded.

RESULTS

- In this cluster-randomized trial, baseline characteristics were similar between the 2 groups of mother–infant pairs in terms of maternal age, education, atopic family history, previous breastfeeding, smoking, Cesarean section, and infant sex.
- Intervention site infants had higher rates of any breastfeeding at 3 m (73% versus 60%; adjusted odds ratio [aOR] 0.52, 95% CI 0.40 to 0.69).
- Infants at BFHI sites had a significant reduction in the risk of ≥1 gastrointestinal tract infections (9.1% versus 13.2%; aOR 0.60; 95% CI, 0.40 to 0.91).
- Improvements in secondary outcomes included other improvements in breastfeeding rates at BFHI sites (exclusively breastfed at 3 months and 6 months, breastfed to any degree at 12 months). Additionally, infants at BFHI sites had a significant reduction in atopic eczema.
- There was no change in respiratory tract infection.

Criticisms and Limitations: It is not possible to conduct an ethical RCT where individual mother–infant pairs are randomly allocated to breastfeed or not. Hence the study design of this cluster-randomized trial focused on support of breastfeeding mothers. It indirectly informs us of the impact of improved breastfeeding rates.

Any trial conducted in a specific healthcare setting will have issues of generalizability. Belarus healthcare and population characteristics differ considerably from other regions of the world. When this trial was conducted (late 1990s), healthcare practices with regard to breastfeeding support (and maternity practices in general) were considered to have been like Western Europe and North America 20 to 30 years previously. However, basic healthcare services and sanitary conditions are very similar, including uncontaminated water supply monitored by public health authorities, and clinics were abundant and readily accessible even in rural areas. This combination of factors enabled the investigators to perform a large and ethical cluster-randomized trial of breastfeeding promotion with adequate generalizability.

Notably, the study did not address the unique needs and challenges of providing breastmilk for the preterm infant, a population that could have even greater benefit with outcomes such as sepsis or necrotizing enterocolitis.

Other Relevant Studies and Information:
- PROBIT emphasizes the impact of staff attitudes and behaviors on breastfeeding success, and its findings resulted in widespread clinical uptake.
- This study (PROBIT I) has formed the basis for further follow-up of 13,889 children representing 85% of the 12 m cohort (PROBIT II) at 6.5 years, (PROBIT III) at 11.5 years, (PROBIT IV) at 16 years. There were no downstream effects on clinically important outcomes, such as growth, blood pressure, or obesity.[3–5]

Summary and Implications: This important and influential trial confirms the beneficial effects that BFHI or similar approaches can have on breastfeeding success. It also demonstrates the beneficial effects of breastmilk exposure in the first year of life.

A CONVERSATION WITH THE TRIALIST: MICHAEL KRAMER

How does your success in using a bundle of practices translate to other healthcare settings?

Difficult to say. Implementation of our experimental intervention was certainly facilitated by the prevailing local culture that has a tradition of "following the rules," i.e., doing what the chief obstetricians and pediatricians asked them to do. In Belarus, we found exactly the same results when we analyzed data according to actual breastfeeding (i.e., "as treated") as when we analyzed by intention to treat ("as randomized"), suggesting very different confounding influences in Belarus than in the West. In particular, the influence of education, income, and lifestyle factors on breastfeeding behavior is probably far weaker in Belarus than in the West. Even if "compliance" with the randomized intervention would have been lower in other populations, the EFFECT of the intervention is unlikely to be different in other settings.

Do you think it likely that promotion of kangaroo mother care (KMC) might act synergistically with BFHI?

There is not so much overlap, I believe. KMC has mostly been studied in preterm and LBW [low birth weight] newborns, whereas PROBIT was restricted to term infants with normal birth weight.

Can you comment on what you hope the future holds for breastfeeding promotion interventions?

Randomized trials of breastfeeding support interventions in women who are obliged (or wish) to return to work after 2–4 months are needed, especially in the Asian setting, where prolonged maternity leaves are extremely rare.

References

1. Kramer MS, Chalmers B, Hodnett ED, et al. Promotion of Breastfeeding Intervention Trial (PROBIT): a randomized trial in the Republic of Belarus. *JAMA.* 2001;285(4):413–20.
2. World Health Organization. *Ten steps to successful breastfeeding.* https://www.who.int/teams/nutrition-and-food-safety/food-and-nutrition-actions-in-health-systems/ten-steps-to-successful-breastfeeding
3. Kramer MS, Matush L, Vanilovich I, et al. Effects of prolonged and exclusive breastfeeding on child height, weight, adiposity, and blood pressure at age 6.5 y: evidence from a large randomized trial. *Am J Clin Nutr.* 2007;86(6):1717–21.
4. Martin RM, Patel R, Kramer MS, et al. Effects of promoting longer-term and exclusive breastfeeding on adiposity and insulin-like growth factor-I at age 11.5 years: a randomized trial. *JAMA.* 2013;309(10):1005–1013.
5. Flohr C, Henderson AJ, Kramer MS, et al. Effect of an intervention to promote breastfeeding on asthma, lung function, and atopic eczema at age 16 years: follow-up of the PROBIT randomized trial. *JAMA Pediatr.* 2018;172(1):e174064.

22

Dextrose Gel for Neonatal Hypoglycemia

The Sugar Babies Trial

ADEL MOHAMED, JYOTSNA SHAH, AND PRAKESH S. SHAH

> "Dextrose gel should be considered for first line management of late pre-term and term hypoglycaemic babies in the first 48 hours after birth."
> —HARRIS ET AL.[1]

Research Question: Is dextrose gel plus feeding more effective than placebo gel plus feeding to resolve neonatal hypoglycemia in at-risk late preterm and term neonates in the first 48 hours (h) of life?

Why Was This Study Done: Hypoglycemia is the most common metabolic disorder of newborns and has been associated with brain injury and adverse neurodevelopmental outcomes. While dextrose gel had been recommended over a decade earlier,[2] there was no trial evidence on its safety and efficacy for the treatment of neonatal hypoglycemia.

Year Study Began: 2008

Study Published: 2013

Study Location: New Zealand (single center)

Who Was Studied: Infants at risk for hypoglycemia (by at least one of the following risk factors: diabetic mother, late prematurity [35 to 36 weeks' gestation], birth weight <2500 g or <10th percentile, birth weight >4500 g or >90th percentile, history of poor feeding) who developed hypoglycemia (defined as a blood glucose <2.6 mmol/L) prior to 48 h of age.

Who was Excluded: Infants with prior treatment for hypoglycemia, serious congenital malformations, life-threatening disorders, or skin abnormalities that prevented continuous glucose monitoring.

How Many Patients: 242. (Of note, 237 were analyzed, as 5 were randomized in error.)

Study Overview: The Sugar Babies trial was a parallel-group, masked RCT (Figure 22.1).

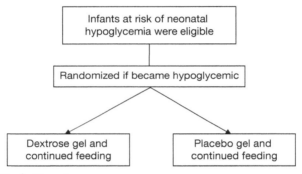

Figure 22.1 Study Overview

What Were the Interventions:
- Infants randomized to the intervention group received 200 mg/kg dextrose gel massaged into the buccal mucosa.
- Infants randomized to the placebo group received identical-appearing 2% carboxymethyl cellulose placebo gel massaged into the buccal mucosa.

Infants from both groups were encouraged to feed after treatment. Blood glucose concentration was measured 30 minutes after gel administration. If the infant remained hypoglycemic or became hypoglycemic at later measurement, the assigned treatment was repeated. Up to 6 doses of gel could be given over a 48-hour period. In a subgroup of neonates, subcutaneous glucose monitoring pumps were inserted to record continuous levels of interstitial glucose concentration for later analysis, but treating clinicians did not have access to these data.

How Long Was Follow-up: 2 weeks

What Were the Endpoints:
Primary Outcome: Treatment failure, defined as a blood glucose <2.6 mmol/L 30 minutes after a second dose of dextrose gel.
Selected secondary outcomes: Admission to the NICU for hypoglycemia; feeding pattern in the first 48 h; frequency of treatment with study gel in the first 48 h; rebound and recurrent hypoglycemia.

Concerns Regarding Bias: The study was at overall low risk of bias.

RESULTS:

- Treatment failure rates were lower for infants receiving dextrose gel than those receiving placebo gel (14% versus 24%; RR 0.57, 95% CI 0.33 to 0.98, $p = 0.04$). Both groups received comparable amounts of study gel (dextrose or placebo), with a median of 2 doses (range 1 to 5) administered in each group ($p = 0.45$).
- Infants in the dextrose gel group were less likely to be admitted to the NICU for hypoglycemia (14% versus 25%; RR 0.54, 95% CI 0.31 to 0.93, $p = 0.03$).
- Feeding patterns were comparable between groups at 48 h; but at 2 weeks of age, fewer babies were formula feeding in the dextrose gel group than in the placebo gel group (4% versus 13%; RR 0.34, 95% CI 0.13 to 0.90, $p = 0.03$).
- Dextrose gel treatment was well tolerated, with no serious adverse effects noted.

Criticisms and Limitations: There are several points of consideration when applying the findings of this well-designed study to clinical care. First, a clinical correlate is lacking, with no information given on how many infants had clinical signs of hypoglycemia. This is an important consideration, especially given that over three-quarters of neonates in the placebo group recovered without treatment. The trial recruited patients at lower risk of prolonged hypoglycemia than anticipated. Treatment failure rates in both groups were lower than assumed for the calculation of the target sample size. Moreover, the difficulty of translating blood glucose values into relevant clinical outcomes is demonstrated here, since no impact of the short-term benefits was observed when 2-year neurodevelopmental outcomes were subsequently reported (See Other Relevant Studies and Information section).

Additionally, while there is clear appeal for further information on the effect of dextrose gel via masked continuous glucose monitoring, the information provided by this study subgroup was difficult to interpret, as these monitors took 1 h to initialize and most episodes of hypoglycemia had already been treated by that point. This reduced the power of these comparisons.

Overall, while this trial provides evidence that may facilitate the treatment of a commonly defined threshold for hypoglycemia, further trial evidence is needed to understand the association between low glucose levels, their time course, and in particular, the longer-term neurologic outcomes.[3]

Other Relevant Studies and Information:
- Two-year outcomes of this trial demonstrated no difference in the neurodevelopmental outcomes of infants randomized to dextrose gel versus those randomized to placebo gel, with frequent rates of neurosensory impairment in both groups (38% versus 34%).[4]
- The recent hPOD trial, which included 2149 infants, did not demonstrate a reduction in NICU admissions with dextrose gel versus placebo, although there was a reduction in hypoglycemia. Feeding patterns were comparable between the 2 groups.[5] Two-year follow-up demonstrated no significant impact with dextrose gel on neurosensory impairment (21% versus 19%).[6]
- The most recent Cochrane review on this topic evaluated dextrose gel initiated within the first 24 h of life and included only hPOD and a smaller initial study by the same group, Pre-hPOD.[7] Meta-analysis of these two RCTs found that oral dextrose gel reduced the risk of treatment for hypoglycemia, but had no impact on receipt of intravenous treatment for hypoglycemia or the separation from the mother for treatment.[8]

Summary and Implications: This randomized controlled trial, conducted at a single center, paved the way for exploring the safety and efficacy of a treatment that had already been introduced to neonatal care. Its results encouraged the use of dextrose gel as the first-line management for neonatal hypoglycemia. Moreover, the study shed light on crucial aspects related to the management of hypoglycemia, such as maternal–infant separation and neurodevelopmental consequences, which are still under investigation.

A CONVERSATION WITH THE TRIALIST: JANE E. HARDING

Oral dextrose gel prevented NICU admissions for hypoglycemia (although did not decrease separation for all reasons). Did you consider tools to measure parent satisfaction regarding this impactful difference? Do you think people underestimate the importance of this treatment, given the success in decreasing NICU admissions for hypoglycemia?

In the Sugar Babies Study, parents reported being satisfied with the use of gel, but we did not further explore which effects in particular were important to them. A subsequent survey of health practitioners involved in maternity care about priorities in management of neonatal hypoglycaemia found that 88% considered separation of mother and baby was important or very important, and 88% considered reduced NICU admissions for hypoglycaemia was important or very important.[1] In addition, the cost savings related to the use of dextrose gel are largely attributable to reducing NICU stay.[2] We are in the process of undertaking qualitative studies to further investigate parental priorities in the management of babies at risk of neonatal hypoglycaemia, which will help inform this question.

1. Liu G, Grigg C, Harding JE. New Zealand practitioners' views about neonatal hypoglycaemia and its management. *J Paediatr Child Health.* 2021;57:1148–1153.
2. Glasgow MJ, Harding JE, Edlin R; Children with Hypoglycemia and Their Later Development (CHYLD) Study Team. Cost analysis of treating neonatal hypoglycemia with dextrose gel. *J Pediatr.* 2018;198: 151–5.

References

1. Harris DL, Weston PJ, Signal M, et al. Dextrose gel for neonatal hypoglycaemia (the Sugar Babies Study): a randomised, double-blind, placebo-controlled trial. *Lancet.* 2013;382(9910):2077–83.
2. D Bourchier, P Weston, P Heron. Hypostop for neonatal hypoglycaemia. *N Z Med J.* 1992;105:22.
3. Marlow N. Treatment of blood glucose concentrations in newborn babies. *Lancet.* 2013;382(9910):2045–6.
4. Harris DL, Alsweiler JM, Ansell JM, et al. Outcome at 2 years after dextrose gel treatment for neonatal hypoglycemia: follow-up of a randomized trial. *J Pediatr.* 2016;170:54–9.
5. Harding JE, Hegarty JE, Crowther CA, et al.; hPOD Study Group. Evaluation of oral dextrose gel for prevention of neonatal hypoglycemia (hPOD): A multicenter, double-blind randomized controlled trial. *PLoS Med.* 2021 Jan 28;18(1):e1003411.

6. Edwards T, Alsweiler JM, Crowther CA, et al. Prophylactic Oral Dextrose Gel and Neurosensory Impairment at 2-Year Follow-up of Participants in the hPOD Randomized Trial. *JAMA*. 2022;327(12):1149–57.

7. Hegarty JE, Harding JE, Gamble GD, et al. Prophylactic oral dextrose gel for newborn babies at risk of neonatal hypoglycaemia: a randomised controlled dose-finding trial (the Pre-hPOD Study). *PLoS Med*. 2016;13(10):e1002155.

8. Edwards T, Liu G, Hegarty JE, et al. Oral dextrose gel to prevent hypoglycaemia in at-risk neonates. *Cochrane Database Syst Rev*. 2021 May 17;5(5):CD012152.

23

Effect of Supplemental Donor Human Milk Compared With Preterm Formula on Neurodevelopment of Very Low Birth Weight Infants at 18 Months

The DoMINO Trial

NICHOLAS D. EMBLETON

"If donor milk is used in a setting with high provision of mother's milk, [neurodevelopment at 18 months of age] should not be considered a treatment goal."

—O'CONNOR ET AL.[1]

Research Question: To determine if nutrient-enriched donor human milk (DHM) compared with preterm formula (PTF), as a supplement to mother's own milk (MOM), reduces neonatal morbidity, supports growth, and improves neurodevelopment in very low birth weight (VLBW) infants.

Why Was This Study Done: Despite widespread global use, prior to this trial, there were very few high-quality, adequately powered studies of DHM and no comparable studies with neurodevelopmental outcome in infancy.

Year Study Began: 2010

Year Study Published: 2016

Study Location: Canada (4 centers)

Who Was Studied: Infants with birth weight <1500 g who were to commence enteral feeding within 7 days of birth and were consented within 96 hours of birth.

Who Was Excluded: Infants with major anomalies, severe birth asphyxia, enrolled in another nutritional study, or who had reasonable potential of transfer to a non-participating unit.

How Many Patients: 363 infants were randomized; 47 were withdrawn or lost to follow-up before discharge and 17 did not have neurodevelopment assessed. Of the 299 assessed for primary outcome, 221 had received an intervention. The remaining 78 infants only received MOM; this was evenly distributed across study arms.

Study Overview: The DoMINO (Donor Milk for Improved Neurodevelopmental Outcomes) study was a parallel-group, masked RCT (Figure 23.1).

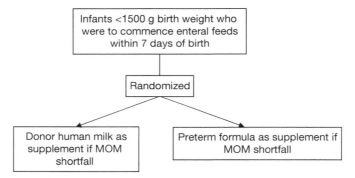

Figure 23.1 Study Overview

What Were the Interventions: Where there was insufficient MOM available to meet infants' enteral intake needs, infants either received DHM or 1 of 2 proprietary PTFs as a supplement.

How Long Was Follow-up: 18 months' CA (18 m)

What Were the Endpoints:
Primary outcome: Cognitive composite score on Bayley Scale of Infant and Toddler Development, Third Edition (BSID-III) at 18 m.

Secondary outcomes: BSID-III language and motor composite scores, a mortality and morbidity index (a dichotomous variable indicating either death or presence of one of a predetermined list of major morbidities considered negatively correlated with provision of human milk (late-onset sepsis, NEC, BPD, and ROP), and growth during feeding intervention.

Concerns Regarding Bias: This study was at overall low risk of bias.

RESULTS

- Over 90% of survivors in both arms underwent neurodevelopmental assessment, and there were no differences in any BSID-III primary or secondary outcomes.
- There were no significant differences in any growth parameters.
- In preplanned analysis, there were fewer cases of NEC stage ≥2 with DHM compared with PTF (1.7% versus 6.6%; $p = 0.02$).
- In post hoc exploratory analysis, more infants receiving DHM compared with PTF had a composite cognitive score of <85, indicative of neuro-impairment (27.2% versus 16.2%; $p = 0.02$).

Criticisms and Limitations: Conducting nutritional trials is challenging, especially across multiple hospital sites, and masking of an intervention such as DHM is especially difficult. At the outset it is impossible to know how much exposure to the intervention the infants may receive, as some may receive none, and others virtually 100%. Using a pragmatic, intention-to-treat methodology is appropriate but means that a significant proportion of the infants undergoing primary outcome assessment were never exposed to the intervention. The authors made multiple a priori assumptions in the calculation of the sample size, estimating 352 infants would be needed. Nonetheless complex post hoc analysis was required, to grapple with potential for confounders. For example, an infant who received all PTF for the first 10 days before maternal supply improved may have a very different risk of NEC to one who initially received all maternal milk and only received PTF starting in the second or third month.

Although differences in BSID were not noted in infants exposed to the intervention, the BSID-III is an insensitive tool, particularly at 18 months. Childhood follow-up is planned.

It is reassuring that there were no significant differences in growth, as DHM is of lower nutrient density than PTF. Some of this can be corrected by the addition of breast milk fortifiers; however, because the components of fortifiers are the same as PTF, any difference in the rate of NEC is unlikely due to bovine protein exposure itself and more likely to reflect benefits of components in DHM such as human milk oligosaccharides (HMOs).[2] While using DHM is standard practice, there may also be considerable variation in concentrations of nutrients and functional components (e.g., HMOs) in different batches of DHM.

Although there was a significant difference in the rate of NEC, it is not clear when NEC occurred or how it related to the trial exposures. It is possible that some cases of NEC occurred prior to exposure to either DHM or PTF. Recognition of NEC stage 2 is not straightforward, with considerable inter-clinician variability; however, the NEC stage $\geq$2 rate of 6.6% in the PTF arm is similar to rates seen in many other units.

Other Relevant Studies and Information:
- A study of similar design and size was conducted in the Netherlands (the Early Nutrition Study) and was also published in 2016.[3] There were no differences in the primary outcome of a composite score of NEC, sepsis, or death. Although critics have argued that this study was of relatively short duration (the first 10 days of life), around 60% of all key events had occurred during that period.
- The most recent Cochrane meta-analysis[4] only identified 4 trials, consisting of <1000 infants in total, that compared use of fortified DHM versus PTF where NEC was reported. Of these, only 3 were published in the last 15 years. The risk of NEC $\geq$2 with use of PTF was of borderline significance (RR 1.64, 95% CI 1.03 to 2.61).

Summary and Implications: The DoMINO trial shows that use of DHM rather than PTF for a shortfall in supply of MOM does not have a significant impact on neurodevelopment at 18 m, and no clearly demonstrable adverse growth effects on preterm infants. It provides some evidence that DHM use may reduce the incidence of NEC; however, a study powered to detect a substantial reduction in NEC (e.g., 5% to 2.5% reduction at 90% power) would require around 2,500 infants. There is not a single published, adequately powered study of an intervention to reduce NEC (including DHM), a disease that has been the scourge of neonatology for more than 40 years, and that remains one of the commonest causes of death and serious disability in this population.

A CONVERSATION WITH THE TRIALIST: DEBORAH O'CONNOR

Future trials of pasteurized donor human milk (PDHM) might focus on other outcomes rather than Bayley scores; can you suggest trial designs that are practical and feasible given the widespread belief that PDHM rather than preterm formula is better for preterm infants?

Trials examining the impact on neurodevelopment of continuing the use of PDHM versus preterm formula as a supplement for very low birth weight (VLBW) infants after 34 weeks, would be worthwhile. Likewise, studies examining the safety and efficacy [of] using PDHM as a supplement for the late preterm infant would be worthwhile.

We know that both the nutrient and bioactive component composition of PDHM differs from parent's own milk. This is due to several factors including the fact that donor milk often consists of mature milk collected several weeks after birth, and at least one extra freeze–thaw cycle and container change in processing. Additionally, PDHM in North America is heat treated (Holder Method, 62.5°C for 30 minutes) to destroy pathogens that could harm a vulnerable infant. A lot of research is going on presently to examine how to improve the quality of donor milk through less harsh processing methods, including nonthermal technologies.

Future studies that compare health outcomes (including neurodevelopment) of VLBW infants fed PDHM processed and nutrient-enriched in new ways over current approaches will be very important.

VLBW infants were randomized to a management strategy that allowed for PDHM supplementation, rather than specifically randomizing infants who required supplementation of mothers' milk. What were the advantages and disadvantages of this approach?

Prior to commencing the trial, we collected feeding data from the recruiting centres to understand the percentage of infants requiring a supplement; this was taken into account in our sample size calculation.

In our high mother's milk use setting, almost all mothers make some attempt to provide their own milk. In order to ensure blinding of all supplemental feeds, we randomized infants within 96 hours of birth. We believe this is important as we don't fully understand the mechanisms of how early feeding impacts health outcomes (e.g., is it the avoidance of cow's milk or the provision of human milk components that is important or both). While a parent's intention to provide exclusively their own milk is a predictor of exclusive parent milk feeding, it is not a precise one.

> *Our methodology allowed us to approach all families in a similar way (including antenatally), enabled prospective data collection from the time of first enteral feeding, and allowed for a built-in reference group of mother's own milk feeders. This reference group is invaluable in the interpretation of findings and in subsequent exploratory analysis in preparation for future studies. The limitation of this approach was, of course, cost. To confirm, the study syringes in our trial did indicate whether they contained mother's own milk or a supplement.*

References

1. O'Connor DL, Gibbins S, Kiss A, et al. Effect of supplemental donor human milk compared with preterm formula on neurodevelopment of very low-birth-weight infants at 18 months: a randomized clinical trial. *JAMA*. 2016 Nov 8;316(18):1897–1905.
2. Masi AC, Embleton ND, Lamb CA, et al. Human milk oligosaccharide DSLNT and gut microbiome in preterm infants predicts necrotising enterocolitis. *Gut*. 2021 Dec;70(12):2273–82.
3. Corpeleijn WE, de Waard M, Christmann V, et al. Effect of donor milk on severe infections and mortality in very low-birth-weight infants: the Early Nutrition Study randomized clinical trial. *JAMA Pediatr*. 2016 Jul 1;170(7):654–61.
4. Quigley M, Embleton ND, McGuire W. Formula versus donor breast milk for feeding preterm or low birth weight infants. *Cochrane Database Syst Rev*. 2019 Jul 19;7:CD002971.

Thermal

24

The Influence of the Thermal Environment Upon the Survival of Newly Born Premature Infants

DAVID OSBORN

"The results of the present study lend support to the long-held view that survival rates of premature infants can be raised by reducing their heat loss."

—SILVERMAN ET AL.[1]

Research Question: In preterm infants in the first 120 hours after birth, does a higher ambient temperature (31.1 to 32.3°C, 88 to 90°F) compared with lower ambient temperature (28.3 to 29.4°C, 83 to 85°F) improve survival to 28 days?

Why Was This Study Done: The authors previously conducted a RCT that showed improved survival of preterm infants nursed in a higher humidity environment.[2] They noted a higher mortality rate in infants with lower body temperatures, and formulated a "normothermic hypothesis." This stated that an ample supply of heat provided to preterm infants will make the smallest metabolic demand and result in increased survival.

Year Study Began: 1956

Year Study Published: 1958

Study Location: United States (single center)

Who Was Studied: Preterm babies <72 hours age, in 3 weight strata (≤1,000 g, 1,001 to 1,500 g, and ≥1,501 g).

Who Was Excluded: No exclusion criteria reported.

How Many Patients: By design, the study did not report a sample size calculation. Instead, paired sequential analysis method determined an a priori stopping rule. Analysis examined only any discrepant survival of the paired infants ("untied" pairs). Stopping was set if boundaries were broached at α = 5% and β = 10%. The final sample was 194 infants, but only 182 were included in the analysis of the main outcome.

Study Overview: This was a parallel-group, unmasked RCT comparing higher and lower incubator temperatures (Figure 24.1). Using a factorial design, infants were also randomized to different doses of tetracycline. The manuscript and this chapter focus on the comparison of incubator temperatures made by collapsing these groups.

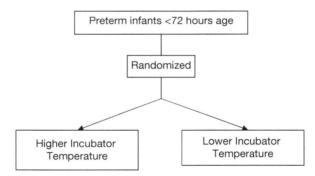

Figure 24.1 Study Overview

What Were the Interventions:
- Infants randomized to the higher incubator temperature group were placed in an incubator set at 31.7°C (89°F), range 31.1 to 32.2°C (88 to 90°F).
- Infants in the lower incubator temperature group were placed in an incubator set at 28.9°C (84°F), range 28.3 to 29.4°C (83 to 85°F).

Both groups had relative humidity set to 80–90%. Infants remained at the set temperature for 120 hours, then were placed at the same weaning temperature and humidity for the rest of their stay.

How Long Was Follow-up: 28 days

What Were the Endpoints:
Primary outcome: Survival to 5 days of age.
Selected secondary outcomes: Survival to 28 days, axillary temperatures, respiratory rates, retraction scores.

Concerns Regarding Bias: The study was at high risk for performance/detection bias, as caregivers were not blinded to the intervention. Additional bias may be present with sequential analysis of paired trial data determining termination of study enrollment, and exclusion of 12 infants (6%) from the analysis.

RESULTS

- The study was terminated when, of 26 "untied" pairs, 20 favored the "normothermic" hypothesis.
- There was a reduction in 5-day mortality in infants in the higher incubator temperature group compared with the lower incubator temperature group (16% versus 32%; RR 0.52, 95% CI 0.30 to 0.90, $p = 0.02$). This difference most pronounced in the lower birth weight strata. *
- There was a reduction in neonatal mortality (to 28 days) in the higher incubator temperature group (22% versus 45%; RR 0.49, 95% CI 0.31 to 0.76, $p = 0.002$). *
- Infants in the higher incubator temperature group had higher axillary temperatures. The infants in the higher incubator temperature group also had slightly higher respiratory rates, but no difference in retraction scores.

*Typical estimates, 95% CI, and *p*-values calculated by chapter authors.

Criticisms and Limitations: Although the stopping rule for this trial was prespecified, paired data were sequentially monitored, increasing the probability of obtaining a statistically significant result, and the stopping rule was at a low statistical probability ($p = 0.05$). Evidence suggests that trials stopped early for benefit systematically overestimate treatment effects, sometimes by a large amount. As an alternative, a threefold approach is recommended: a low P-value as the threshold for stopping at the time of interim analyses, not to look before a sufficiently large number of events has accrued, and continuation of enrollment and follow-up for a further period.[3]

The hypothesis was to provide an ample supply of heat to preterm infants to make the smallest metabolic demand in the higher incubator temperature group. However, especially in the lower weight strata, infants in this group would today be considered hypothermic (1000 to 1500 g: mean 36.0°C ± 0.7 SD; and <1001 g: 33.7°C ± 1.5).[4]

Other Relevant Studies and Information:
- Silverman et al. subsequently estimated that minimal rates of oxygen consumption in very low birth weight infants occur when abdominal skin temperature is regulated at 36–37°C ("the neutral thermal zone").[5]
- A systematic review found that use of servo-controlled incubators with skin temperature set at 36.5°C decreases neonatal mortality.[6]
- Current European Consensus Guidelines on the Management of Respiratory Distress Syndrome recommend core temperature should be maintained between 36.5 and 37.5°C at all times.[7]

Summary and Implications: This trial represents one of a series of path-breaking trials performed by Silverman and colleagues that largely introduced the concept of RCTs to identify critical needs of preterm infants. This trial of higher versus lower incubator temperature for preterm infants in the first 5 days provided good evidence that targeting a higher temperature (albeit not in the "neutral thermal zone") reduced mortality. This formed the basis for subsequent research providing evidence for targeting a skin temperature 36.5°C.

A CONVERSATION WITH THE TRIALIST: WRITINGS OF BILL SILVERMAN

Dr. Silverman is considered to be the "father of neonatal intensive care." Silverman urged physicians to seek evidence for the myriad of interventions introduced into neonatal care. His work in promoting randomized trials is epitomized in his trials delineating the role of oxygen in ROP (then called retrolental fibroplasia) and the thermal environment including his trials of humidity and the trial of temperature control discussed in this chapter.

No words can represent Silverman better than his own, and he fortunately left extensive writings on his experiences. On the evolution of this trial on temperature control he wrote: "In 'dredging' through the records [of a previous trial on humidity], we found a small but consistent decrease in body temperature among infants reared in 'low humidity' (30%–60% relative humidity). It seemed very unlikely to us that slightly low body temperature was responsible for an increase in mortality: for more than 20 years, incubator temperatures in America had been intentionally set to maintain relatively low but steady body temperature . . . based on the findings in a prolonged observational study. . . . In March 1956, we began a trial comparing first-five-day mortality among infants housed in incubators maintained at 2 contrasting levels of ambient temperature. . . In February 1957, a pre-determined 'decision-line' was crossed, indicating that lower mortality was associated with the warmer incubators."[1]

1. Silverman WA. Personal reflections on lessons learned from randomized trials involving newborn infants, 1951 to 1967. *Clin Trials.* 2004;1:179–84.

References

1. Silverman WA, Fertig JW, Berger AP. The influence of the thermal environment upon the survival of newly born premature infants. *Pediatrics.* 1958;22:876–86.
2. Silverman WA, Balnc WA. The effect of humidity on survival of newly born premature infants. *Pediatrics.* 1957;20:477–86.
3. Bassler D, Montori VM, Briel M, et al. Early stopping of randomized clinical trials for overt efficacy is problematic. *J Clinl Epidemiol.* 2008;61:241–6.
4. World Health Organization. (1997) Thermal Protection of the Newborn: A Practical Guide. https://apps.who.int/iris/bitstream/handle/10665/63986/WHO_RHT_MSM_97.2.pdf
5. Silverman WA, Sinclair JC, Agate FJ, Jr. The oxygen cost of minor changes in heat balance of small newborn infants. *Acta Paediatr Scand.* 1966;55:294–300.
6. Sinclair JC. Servo-control for maintaining abdominal skin temperature at 36C in low birth weight infants. *Cochrane Database Syst Rev.* 2002;1:CD001074.
7. Sweet DG, Carnielli V, Greisen G, et al. European Consensus Guidelines on the Management of Respiratory Distress Syndrome: 2022 Update. *Neonatology.* 2023;120(1):3–23.

25

Kangaroo Mother Versus Traditional Care for Newborn Infants <2000 Grams

SRINIVAS MURKI

"These results show that KMC is a safe approach to the care of clinically stable LBW infants. Our findings provide the necessary scientific support to a method that is already incorporated in the care of LBW infants at many hospitals around the world and at different levels of care."

—CHARPAK ET AL.[1]

Research Question: In infants with birth weights <2000 g who have overcome major adaptation problems to extrauterine life and are eligible for admission to a minimal care unit, does kangaroo mother care (KMC), in comparison with traditional care, affect mortality and growth at 40 to 41 weeks' postmenstrual age (PMA)?

Why Was This Study Done: Limited evidence on KMC with all its components (early discharge, skin-to-skin contact, breastfeeding) was available prior to this study, although the practice was already incorporated at many hospitals, of varying levels of care.

Year Study Began: 1993

Year Study Published: 1997

Study Location: Colombia

Who Was Studied: Infants with birth weight <2000 g and eligible for admission to a "minimal care unit," where mothers would receive training in KMC.

Who Was Excluded: Infants with life-threatening or major malformations, or early-detected major conditions arising from perinatal problems (severe hypoxic–ischemic encephalopathy, pulmonary hypertension). Families who were unable to comply with the study protocol were also excluded.

How Many Patients: 746

Study Overview: This trial was a parallel group, unmasked, stratified block RCT (Figure 25.1).

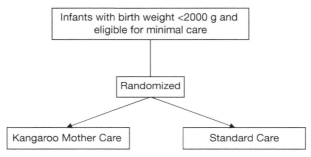

Figure 25.1 Study Overview

What Were the Interventions:
- Mother–infant dyads in the KMC group were transferred from the birth hospital upon randomization, to receive training in KMC at a separate hospital prior to discharge to home. Once home, these babies were kept 24 hours a day in a strict upright position, in skin-to-skin contact, firmly attached to the mother's chest. Babies were breastfed regularly, and premature formula supplements were administered to guarantee adequate weight gain if necessary. Infants remained in the kangaroo position until they no longer accepted it by demonstrating discomfort, pushing out limbs, and crying and fussing when mothers tried to return them to the upright position.
- Infants in the control group received standard care, including incubator care until they established mature thermoregulation and appropriate weight gain. Infants were discharged according to existing hospital practice (usually not before reaching a weight of 1700 g). At the time

of the study, practice at the study NICU included restricted parental access to their infants.

How Long Was Follow-up: 40 to 41 weeks' PMA

What Were the Endpoints:
Primary outcome: Mortality and growth.
Selected secondary outcomes: Length of hospital stay, infection, breastfeeding.

Concerns Regarding Bias: This study was at high risk for performance/detection bias, as caregivers were not blinded to the intervention. Use of fixed blocked randomization could have allowed prediction of future assignments in this unmasked trial. While consent was obtained after randomization and only for those assigned to the KMC group, none of the mothers randomized to KMC declined consent.

RESULTS

- The mortality did not differ between the 2 groups (relative risk 0.59, 95% confidence interval 0.22 to 1.6), and growth indices were similar.
- After adjusting for weight at eligibility, KMC resulted in shorter hospital stays by an average of 1.1 day; this difference was larger in infants born <1200 g.
- Rates of infection were similar between groups, as were rates of exclusive and partial breastfeeding.

Criticisms and Limitations: Several considerations for the interpretation of these study findings are worth noting. First, given the time required to train parents in KMC prior to discharge to home, nearly 80% of the infants in both groups required equal time from randomization until hospital discharge. The duration of hospital stay was lowest for the infants in the KMC group when birth weight was <1500 grams, but these infants formed only 20% of the total study population. Secondly, although the study mandated 24/7 skin-to-skin contact in the KMC group, the exact duration of KMC in hours and days after randomization is not reported in the study. Finally, in the current context, important elements of the "standard care" provided to the control group (a minimal hospital discharge weight criteria and restriction of family entry to NICU) are now less commonly employed than at the time of the study.

Other Relevant Studies and Information:

- In a meta-analysis of 8 RCTs involving a total of 1736 infants, study participants who received KMC after stabilization had fewer deaths than those who received standard care in an incubator or a radiant warmer (3.2% versus 5.3%; risk difference −0.02, 95% CI −0.04 to − 0.00). Additionally, infants who received KMC had fewer infections, higher rates of exclusive breastfeeding, and better weight gain.[2]
- World Health Organization (WHO) guidelines currently recommend that KMC start immediately after birth, without any initial period in an incubator. [3]
- A recent RCT evaluated the timing of KMC in infants with birth weights between 1000 and 1799 g and showed that initiation of continuous KMC soon after birth improved neonatal survival by 25% as compared with KMC initiated after stabilization.[4]
- This publication presented the primary results for a trial designed to follow infants through the first year of life, with subsequent publication confirming persistent beneficial effects of KMC on mortality and improved growth at 1 year.[5] The study team continued to follow this cohort through 20 years of age, demonstrating social and behavioral protective effects at 20 years.[6]

Summary and Implications: This trial provided early evidence for a practice that had already been incorporated at many centers but not properly evaluated. It contributed to a subsequently growing body of evidence that KMC is safe and beneficial to LBW infants, as well as to an evolving model for better and more integrated support of the mother–baby dyad.

A FEW WORDS FROM THE EDITOR

The study of Charpak and colleagues set into motion an expansive research effort to evaluate kangaroo mother care (KMC), mostly set in low- and middle-income countries. Meta-analysis of 8 trials and the more recent RCT evaluating the timing of KMC in moderately preterm infants have demonstrated improved neonatal survival.[2] The World Health Organization has recently modified their recommendations to advise that KMC should start immediately after birth, without any initial period in an incubator.[3] The guideline acknowledges that KMC is not just about snuggling your baby; changes need to be made in the organization of care, including the infrastructure, equipment, supplies, and staff training necessary to support both the mother and preterm infant.

Will these recommendations also be incorporated as the standard of care in higher-income countries? Even if we do not see a decrease in mortality in these settings, one can hardly argue with the great benefits that will accrue to families who experience this greater engagement with their child.

—Roger Soll

References

1. Charpak N, Ruiz-Peláez JG, Figueroa de CZ, et al. Kangaroo mother versus traditional care for newborn infants. *Pediatrics*. 1997;100:682–8.
2. Conde-Agudelo A, Díaz-Rossello JL. Kangaroo mother care to reduce morbidity and mortality in low birthweight infants. *Cochrane Database Syst Rev*. 2016;8:CD002771.
3. World Health Organization. WHO recommendations for care of the preterm or low-birth-weight infant. 2022 (https://www.who.int/publications/i/item/9789240058262)
4. WHO Immediate KMC Study Group, Arya S, Naburi H, et al. Immediate "Kangaroo Mother Care" and survival of infants with low birth weight. *N Engl J Med*. 2021;384(21):2028–38.
5. Charpak N, Ruiz-Pelaez JG, Figueroa de CZ, et al. A randomized, controlled trial of kangaroo mother care: results of follow-up at 1 year of corrected age. *Pediatrics*. 2001;108(5):1072–79.
6. Charpak N, Tessier R, Ruiz JG. Twenty-year follow-up of kangaroo mother care versus traditional care. *Pediatrics*. 2017;139(1):e20162063.

Infectious Disease / Immunology

26

Palivizumab, a Humanized Respiratory Syncytial Virus Monoclonal Antibody, Reduces Hospitalization From Respiratory Syncytial Virus Infection in High-Risk Infants

The IMpact-RSV Trial

BRIAN CHRISTOPHER KING

"Monthly intramuscular administration of palivizumab is safe and effective for prevention of serious RSV illness in premature children and those with BPD."

—THE IMPACT-RSV STUDY GROUP[1]

Research Question: Does prophylactic monthly administration of palivizumab, a humanized monoclonal antibody targeting the respiratory syncytial virus (RSV), versus placebo in high-risk infants safely reduce the incidence of hospitalization due to RSV over 150 days?

Why Was This Study Done: RSV is a leading cause of respiratory illness in high-risk infants. Prior to palivizumab, RSV prophylaxis could only be achieved using RSV-IGIV, which was an infusion requiring intravenous access.[2]

Year Study Began: 1996

Year Study Published: 1998

Study Location: United States (119 centers), United Kingdom (11 centers), Canada (9 centers)

Who Was Studied: Infants ≤35 weeks' gestational age (GA) and ≤6 months old; or infants ≤24 months with BPD requiring ongoing medical therapy.

Who Was Excluded: Infants undergoing a prolonged hospitalization (>30 days) at the time of recruitment or those already requiring mechanical ventilation; with congenital heart disease (except a patent ductus arteriosus or an uncomplicated septal defect); active or recent RSV infection; known hepatic or renal dysfunction, seizure disorder, immunodeficiency, allergy to immunoglobulin G (IgG) products; receipt of RSV immune globulin within the prior 3 months,; prior receipt of palivizumab or other monoclonal antibodies, or a life expectancy of <6 months.

How Many Patients: 1502—Randomized in a 2:1 ratio (2 treatments to 1 placebo).

Study Overview: Impact-RSV was a parallel-group, masked, RCT (Figure 26.1).

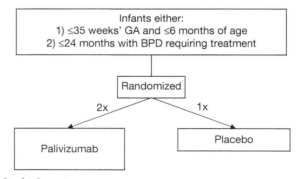

Figure 26.1 Study Overview

What Were the Interventions:
- Infants randomized to treatment received intramuscular (IM) injections of palivizumab (15 mg/kg) every 30 days for a total of 5 doses.
- Infants randomized to placebo received an equal volume of identically appearing placebo.

Interventions were continued for one RSV season.

How Long Was Follow-up: 150 days from randomization (30 days after the last scheduled injection)

What Were the Endpoints:
Primary outcome: RSV hospitalization [defined as a positive RSV antigen test during a hospitalization either for respiratory illness or for other reasons but with evidence of lower respiratory tract illness/infection (LRI)].
Selected secondary outcomes: Duration of hospitalization, total days of increased supplemental oxygen, moderate/severe respiratory illness, mechanical ventilation, duration in the ICU.

Concerns Regarding Bias: The study was at overall low risk of bias. However, the fact that the lead statistician was an employee of the pharmaceutical sponsor could be considered a potential source of bias.

RESULTS

- Monthly palivizumab injections led to a 55% relative reduction in RSV hospitalizations (4.8% versus 10.6%; 95% CI 0.38 to 0.72, p <0.001). Reductions were observed in both subgroups of children (39% reduction in infants with BPD [95% CI 0.20 to 0.58, p = 0.038], 78% reduction in preterm infants [95% CI 0.66 to 9.0, p <0.001]) and across all gestational ages.
- Three percent of placebo patients and 1.3% of palivizumab recipients had RSV ICU admissions (p = 0.026).
- Monthly palivizumab injections reduced total RSV hospital days per 100 children (36.4 versus 62.3; p <0.001), days with increased oxygen (30.3 versus 50.6; p <0.001), and days with an increased LRI score (47.7 versus 29.6; p <0.001).
- There was no difference between the number of reported adverse events in each group (11% palivizumab, 10% placebo), and discontinuation of treatment due to adverse events was rare (0.3%).

Criticisms and Limitations: While a 55% relative reduction in hospitalizations is impressive, the number needed to treat to prevent one hospitalization is estimated to be 17 from the trial results, with a 95% confidence interval up to 36; which in especially vulnerable infants such as BPD is as high as 424. Combining

this with the overall short hospitalizations and uncertain reduction in severe illness or death highlights potential uncertainties in benefit on the societal level.
Indeed, implementation of palivizumab prophylaxis worldwide has been controversial due to questions regarding cost-effectiveness.[3] There was no prospectively
designed economic evaluation alongside the IMpact-RSV trial, and subsequent
economic evaluations have provided inconsistent results.[4,5]

While the primary outcome of a hospitalization secondary to RSV is clinically
significant, it does not completely capture the morbidity of RSV during a single
season, which can also include increased utilization of healthcare resources outside of the hospital. In addition, the study did not address whether continued
prophylaxis during subsequent seasons continues to provide similar protection.
RSV infection may also be associated with long-term morbidity in children (e.g.,
asthma and allergy), and the follow-up period for this study was not able to address those risks.

The authors' decision to include a broad range of infants with very different
baseline risks of RSV hospitalization is notable as an approach more common in
trials with commercial sponsorship, for label intent. The low threshold for treatment used by the study may limit generalizability, as the neonatal community
works to define the optimal population for this treatment.

Other Relevant Studies and Information:
- IM injections with palivizumab made RSV prophylaxis much more
  accessible, replacing the previous prophylactic infusion approach that
  required several hours of administration time and repeated intravenous
  access.
- A similarly designed trial was conducted in infants with congenital heart
  disease (CHD), which showed a 45% reduction in RSV hospitalizations
  ($p = 0.003$), as well as reductions in RSV hospital days and days
  requiring supplemental oxygen.[6]
- The most recent Cochrane review evaluated 5 studies (including this
  one), with a total of 3343 infants. It found that palivizumab reduces
  hospitalization due to RSV infection at 2-year follow-up (RR 0.44, 95%
  CI 0.30 to 0.64; high certainty evidence).[5]
- Although IMpact-RSV broke new ground in showing the effectiveness
  of passive immunization for the prevention of RSV infection, a next
  generation of monoclonal antibody prophylaxis—nirsevimab—that is
  required only once per season has been shown to be efficacious,[7] and
  is being incorporated into routine care for all newborns in the United
  States, as available.
- Results from IMpact-RSV, as well as the trial in infants with CHD
  described earlier in this chapter, have been the primary source of

efficacy data for national guidelines on RSV prophylaxis.[8] Due to the broad gestational age range included and uncertainties regarding cost-effectiveness, and the availability of newer products, there has been significant variation in guideline recommendations for different populations in different settings.[9,10]

Summary and Implications: The IMpact-RSV trial demonstrated that monthly prophylactic injections of palivizumab significantly reduce the burden of RSV hospitalization in preterm infants and infants with BPD. No differences in the critical outcome of ICU admissions or use of mechanical ventilation were noted. This trial provided the bulk of evidence to support clinical guidelines in many countries around the world recommending RSV prophylaxis for preterm infants, though there continues to be controversy regarding the ideal population.

A FEW WORDS FROM THE EDITOR

In the Impact-RSV study, prophylactic monthly injections of palivizumab, a monoclonal antibody targeting RSV, led to a 55% reduction in RSV-related hospitalizations; however, even in this high-risk population, rehospitalization occurs in only 10% of control infants. Importantly, admission to pediatric intensive care, a more concerning clinical outcome, is less common (seen in only 3% of control infants) and was not significantly impacted by treatment, leading to discussions not only of efficacy, but also of cost-effectiveness, with numbers needed to treat rising to the hundreds of infants.

As we have emerged from our COVID-19 precautions, a bitter irony is that we found ourselves facing a second wave of serious respiratory viral illness caused by RSV in otherwise low-risk infants and children.[1] Other strategies that will prevent RSV-related disease, including vaccination of pregnant women and both term and preterm infants, are now underway and may provide a simpler and more universal strategy to prevent this illness in a broad population of infants in diverse settings worldwide.[2]

—Roger Soll

1. Li Y, Wang X, Cong B, et al. Understanding the potential drivers for respiratory syncytial virus rebound during the coronavirus disease 2019 pandemic. *J Infect Dis.* 2022;225(6):957–64.
2. Kampmann B, Madhi SA, Munjal I, et al.; MATISSE Study Group. Bivalent prefusion F vaccine in pregnancy to prevent RSV illness in infants. *N Engl J Med.* 2023;388(16):1451–64.

References

1. The IMpact-RSV Study Group. Palivizumab, a humanized respiratory syncytial virus monoclonal antibody, reduces hospitalization from respiratory syncytial virus infection in high-risk infants. *Pediatrics.* 1998;102(3):531–37.

2. Connor E. Reduction of respiratory syncytial virus hospitalization among premature infants and infants with bronchopulmonary dysplasia using respiratory syncytial virus immune globulin prophylaxis. *Pediatrics.* 1997;99(1):93–99.

3. Embleton ND, Harkensee C, Mckean MC. Palivizumab for preterm infants. Is it worth it? *Arch Dis Child Fetal Neonatal Ed.* 2005;90(4):F286–9.

4. Mac S, Sumner A, Duchesne-Belanger S, et al. Cost-effectiveness of palivizumab for respiratory syncytial virus: a systematic review. *Pediatrics.* 2019 May;143(5):e20184064.

5. Garegnani L, Styrmisdóttir L, Roson Rodriguez P, et al. Palivizumab for preventing severe respiratory syncytial virus (RSV) infection in children. *Cochrane Database Syst Rev.* 2021;11:CD013757.

6. Feltes TF, Cabalka AK, Meissner HC, et al. Palivizumab prophylaxis reduces hospitalization due to respiratory syncytial virus in young children with hemodynamically significant congenital heart disease. *J Pediatr.* 2003;143(4):532–40.

7. Hammit LL, Dagan R, Yuan Y, et al.; MELODY Study Group. Nirsevimab for prevention of RSV in healthy late-preterm and term infants. *N Engl J Med.* 2022;386(9):837–46.

8. Brady MT, Byington CL, Davies HD, et al. Updated guidance for palivizumab prophylaxis among infants and young children at increased risk of hospitalization for respiratory syncytial virus infection. *Pediatrics.* 2014;134(2):415–20.

9. UK Health Security Agency. Chapter 27a. Respiratory syncytial virus. In: The Green Book: Immunisation Against Infectious Disease. Chapter last updated 2015. Accessible at https://www.gov.uk/government/collections/immunisation-against-infectious-disease-the-green-book

10. American Academy of Pediatrics. Nirsevimab Administration. https://www.aap.org/en/patient-care/respiratory-syncytial-virus-rsv-prevention/nirsevimab-administration/ Last updated 11/03/2023.

27

Probiotic Effects on Late-Onset Sepsis in Very Preterm Infants

DEENA THOMAS AND M. JEEVA SHANKAR

"The probiotics *B. infantis, S. thermophilus,* and *B. lactis* significantly reduced NEC of Bell stage 2 or more in very preterm infants, but not definite late-onset sepsis or mortality."

—JACOBS ET AL.[1]

Research Question: Does administration of a combination of 3 probiotic strains (*Bifidobacterium infantis, Streptococcus thermophilus,* and *Bifidobacterium lactis*), versus placebo, to very preterm infants reduce the incidence of culture-positive late-onset sepsis before discharge or 40 weeks' PMA?

Why Was This Study Done: At the time of this trial, mounting evidence suggested that different probiotic strains reduce the risks of NEC and all-cause mortality. However, the impact on late-onset sepsis was unclear, with evidence limited to small trials with inconsistent definitions of late-onset sepsis.

Year Study Began: 2007

Year Study Published: 2013

Study Location: Australia (10 centers), New Zealand (2 centers)

Who Was Studied: Infants born <32 weeks' gestation and weighing <1500 g at birth within 72 hours of birth.

Who Was Excluded: Infants with major congenital malformations or chromosomal anomalies, those likely to die within 72 hours of birth, or infants whose mothers received non-dietary probiotic supplements.

How Many Patients: 1099

Study Overview: This trial was a parallel-group, masked RCT (Figure 27.1).

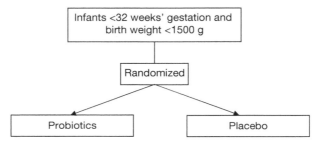

Figure 27.1 Study Overview

What Were the Interventions:
- Infants randomized to the probiotics group received a combination of 3 probiotics (*Bifidobacterium infantis BB-02, Streptococcus thermophilus TH-4*, and *Bifidobacterium lactis BB-12*) with a total of 1×10^9 organisms per 1.5 g in a maltodextrin base. This was chosen because it was commercially available and had been previously tested.
- Infants randomized to the placebo group received 1.5 g of maltodextrin—identical in color and texture to the probiotic powder.
- Daily doses were adjusted according to the volume of milk feeds received, and the interventions were held when infants did not receive any milk feeds.

How Long Was Follow-up: 40 weeks' PMA or discharge, whichever was earlier.

What Were the Endpoints:
Primary outcome: Definite late-onset sepsis, defined as a first episode >48 hours after birth or a subsequent episode occurring ≥72 hours after cessation of antibiotics; with a pathogen isolated from blood, urine, or cerebrospinal fluid; prompting antibiotic treatment for ≥5 days.

Selected secondary outcomes: Clinical late-onset sepsis (negative blood culture, but with elevated C-reactive protein or elevated immature-to-total neutrophil ratio, prompting antibiotic treatment for ≥5 days), mortality, NEC (Bell stage ≥2), or common morbidities of very preterm infants (including PDA, IVH, ROP).

Concerns Regarding Bias: The overall risk of bias was low, and there was no industry funding.

RESULTS

- There was no difference in the risk of definite late-onset sepsis (13.1% versus 16.2% in the probiotic and placebo groups, respectively; RR 0.81, 95% CI 0.61 to 1.08, $p = 0.16$).
- Subgroup analysis revealed a significant reduction in definite late-onset sepsis in infants born ≥28 weeks' gestation (5.5.% versus 10.8%; RR 0.51, 95% CI 0.29 to 0.88, $p = 0.01$).
- Consistent with prior studies, there was a significant reduction in the incidence of NEC in the probiotic group (2.0% versus 4.4%; RR 0.46, 95% CI 0.23 to 0.93, $p = 0.03$). However, rates of NEC were low, and as the authors state, caution in extrapolation is needed. This meant that in this population, the number of very preterm infants that needed to be treated to prevent one additional case of NEC was 43 (95% CI 23 to 333).
- There were no differences in the risks of clinical late-onset sepsis, mortality, or common morbidities between the 2 groups.
- None of the infants developed definite sepsis with any of the probiotic strains used in the study.
- More than 95% of enrolled infants in both groups received breast milk; more than half of them were exclusively breastfed at discharge.

Criticism and Limitations: For their sample size estimation, the authors assumed a definite late-onset sepsis risk of 23% in the control group. However, the observed control group event rate in this study cohort was only 16%. This lower-than-expected risk of sepsis may have reduced the statistical power. Interestingly, the study demonstrated a significant reduction in the incidence of NEC, a much rarer event than late-onset sepsis (4.4% in the placebo group). Coupled with the difference in the potential effect sizes between late-onset sepsis and NEC (19% versus 54% relative reduction), one could hypothesize that the beneficial effects of probiotics are more pronounced at the local (i.e., gut) rather than the systemic level. A few other studies using different probiotic strains demonstrated similarly discordant results between these 2 outcomes.[2,3]

The lack of benefit on mortality, late-onset sepsis, and morbidities other than NEC preclude definitive conclusions about the utility of this probiotic combination. Even for NEC, the precision for the estimate of the treatment benefit was poor: at least 23, but up to 333, very preterm infants may have to be treated with probiotics to prevent one additional case. NICUs with a very low baseline prevalence of severe NEC are unlikely to find value in the intervention. Indeed, a 2016 survey of 500 NICUs in the United States found that only 14% of the units used routine probiotics in very low birth weight infants.[4]

Other Relevant Studies and Information:

- At the time of publication, this was the largest RCT of probiotics for very preterm infants.
- A Cochrane review suggested that probiotics might reduce the risk of NEC, mortality, and late-onset sepsis in very preterm or VLBW infants.[5] However, the sensitivity analysis that included only the 16 trials at low risk of bias (which included the current trial) did not find any effect on mortality or late-onset sepsis.
- The position paper by the European Society for Pediatric Gastroenterology Hepatology and Nutrition (ESPGHAN) Committee on Nutrition and ESPGHAN working group for Probiotics and Prebiotics made a conditional recommendation (with low certainty of evidence) to provide either the combination of the 3 probiotics used in this trial or *Lactobacillus rhamnosus* GG for reducing NEC.[6]
- In contrast, the Committee on Fetus and Newborn, American Academy of Pediatrics (AAP) recommends against routinely prescribing probiotics to ELBW infants, given the conflicting data on the safety and efficacy of probiotics.[7] The Committee stressed the need to develop pharmaceutical-grade probiotics that could be rigorously evaluated in RCTs for safety and efficacy.
- Unfortunately, the optimal strain(s), dose, and duration of the probiotics are unknown even after enrolling more than 10,000 infants in more than 50 trials across the globe.

Summary and Implications: This trial revealed no beneficial effects of probiotics on definite late-onset sepsis and mortality but reported a significant reduction in the risk of NEC in very preterm infants. There is an urgent need for well-designed, large, head-to-head comparison trials of different strains and combinations to identify the optimal probiotic strain(s).

A FEW WORDS FROM THE EDITOR

Few interventions in neonatal perinatal medicine have been more extensively studied than the use of probiotic agents to prevent necrotizing enterocolitis. Yet probiotics are routinely used in only 17% of neonatal intensive care units in the United States.[1] Meta-analysis of over 50 trials suggests a meaningful reduction in NEC, but concern has been voiced over methodological issues and potential publication bias. In a review of data from 807 US NICUs in the Vermont Oxford Network, probiotic adoption was associated with lower NEC risk but not lower risk of sepsis or mortality among VLBW neonates.[1] Although evidence is accumulating in support of probiotic use, there are many issues that remain, including choice of probiotic agents and regulatory hurdles.

—Roger Soll

1. Agha L, Staiger D, Brown C, et al. Association of hospital adoption of probiotics with outcomes among neonates with very low birth weight. *JAMA Health Forum.* 2023 May 5;4(5):e230960.

References

1. Jacobs SE, Tobin JM, Opie GF, et al.; ProPrems Study Group. Probiotic effects on late-onset sepsis in very preterm infants: a randomized controlled trial. *Pediatrics.* 2013;132:1055–62.
2. Dilli D, Aydin B, Fettah ND, et al. The propre-save study: effects of probiotics and prebiotics alone or combined on necrotizing enterocolitis in very low birth weight infants. *J Pediatr.* 2015;166:545–51.
3. Lin HC, Hsu CH, Chen HL, et al. Oral probiotics prevent necrotizing enterocolitis in very low birth weight preterm infants: a multicenter, randomized, controlled trial. *Pediatrics.* 2008;122(4):693–700.
4. Viswanathan S, Lau C, Akbari H, et al. Survey and evidence based review of probiotics used in very low birth weight preterm infants within the United States. *J Perinatol.* 2016;36:1106–11.
5. Sharif S, Meader N, Oddie SJ, et al. Probiotics to prevent necrotising enterocolitis in very preterm or very low birth weight infants. *Cochrane Database Syst Rev.* 2020;(10):CD005496.
6. van den Akker CHP, van Goudoever JB, Shamir R, et al. Probiotics and preterm infants: a position paper by the European Society for Paediatric Gastroenterology Hepatology and Nutrition Committee on Nutrition and the European Society for Paediatric Gastroenterology Hepatology and Nutrition Working Group for Probiotics and Prebiotics. *J Pediatr Gastroenterol Nutr.* 2020;70:664–80.
7. Poindexter B; Committee on Fetus and Newborn. Use of probiotics in preterm infants. *Pediatrics.* 2021;147:e2021051485.

28

Valganciclovir for Symptomatic Congenital Cytomegalovirus Disease

The VGCV Trial

LI MA

"Treating symptomatic congenital CMV disease with valganciclovir for 6 months, as compared with 6 weeks, did not improve hearing in the short term but appeared to improve hearing and developmental outcomes modestly in the longer term."

—KIMBERLIN ET AL.[1]

Research Question: For infants with symptomatic congenital cytomegalovirus (CMV), is a 6-month course versus a 6-week course of oral valganciclovir superior in maintaining hearing in the better ear from baseline to 6 months?

Why Was This Study Done: Earlier work from this group demonstrated that a 6-week course of intravenous ganciclovir improves audiologic outcomes at 6 months for infants with symptomatic congenital cytomegalovirus disease.[2] However, effects were observed to wane over time. Additionally, oral valganciclovir (the prodrug of ganciclovir) had become a treatment option,[3] with dosing based on pharmacodynamics reported by this group.[4]

Year Study Began: 2008

Year Study Published: 2015

Study Location: United States, United Kingdom (31 centers)

Who Was Studied: Neonates with symptomatic congenital CMV; and a gestational age of ≥32 weeks, an age of ≤30 days, and a weight of ≥1800 g at initiation of therapy.

Who Was Excluded: Infants with i) expected imminent demise; ii) poor gastrointestinal and kidney function; iii) administration of other antiviral agents, immune globulin, or other investigational drugs; or iv) mothers who were HIV positive, or receiving other antiviral agents.

How Many Patients: This study was powered on 74 infants with complete follow-up, to detect an effect size of 0.169 from the null value of 0.5. However, only 68 of the 96 enrolled infants completed all follow-up assessments at 24 months.

Study Overview: The VGCV (Valganciclovir) trial was a parallel-group, masked RCT (Figure 28.1).

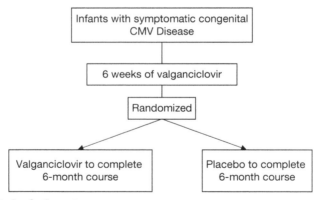

Figure 28.1 Study Overview

What Were the Study Interventions: All participants received standard care oral valganciclovir (at a dose of 16 mg per kilogram of body weight, twice daily) for 6 weeks.

- Infants randomized to 6 months of valganciclovir then received an additional 4.5 months of this regimen, adjusted monthly for growth.
- Infants randomized to placebo then received 4.5 months of a placebo medication.

How Long Was Follow-up: 6 months, 12 months, and 24 months

What Were the Endpoints:
Primary outcome: Change in hearing in the better ear ("best-ear") assessments between baseline and 6 months.
Selected secondary outcomes: Changes in total-ear and best-ear hearing assessments, neurodevelopmental outcomes, whole blood viral load, adverse events related to valganciclovir therapy.

Concerns Regarding Bias: This study was at high risk of bias due to loss of follow-up (attrition rate >30%).

RESULTS

- Change in best-ear hearing at 6 months was not different between the 6-month and 6-week group (adjusted odds ratio [aOR] 1.75, 95% CI 0.69 to 4.43).
- With regard to secondary outcomes, total-ear hearing was more likely to be improved or to remain normal at 12 months in the 6-month group than in the 6-week group (aOR 3.04, 95% CI 1.26 to 7.35), and this benefit was maintained at 24 months (aOR 2.61, 95% CI 1.05 to 6.43).
- Compared with the 6-week group, better neurodevelopmental scores at 24 months were found in 6-month group on the language-composite component and the receptive-communication scale of the Bayley Scales of Infant and Toddler Development, Third Edition.
- Lower viral load was associated with better hearing outcomes at 6, 12, and 24 months in the 6-month group, but not in the 6-week group.
- There was no significant difference in the occurrence of adverse events between the 2 groups; of note, grade 3 or 4 neutropenia occurred in 19% of participants during the first 6 weeks (This was decreased from 63% of ganciclovir-treated patients in the group's earlier study.[2]).

Criticisms and Limitations: CMV is a relatively rare disease, and therefore a randomized trial of therapies is challenging, requiring participation of many centers. The small sample size of the study decreased the power of its findings, importantly of the subgroup assessments stratified by CNS (central nervous system) involvement at baseline, prematurity, or age at initiation of antiviral therapy.

The primary outcome findings are likely to be the most robust, but the a priori secondary outcomes are important. To guard against inadvertent significance being found by chance, a P-value of <0.0071 was needed to retain statistical significance for neurodevelopmental outcomes. This seems a reasonable approach and strengthens the findings; however, the secondary nature of the findings warrants replication.

Eligible participants in the trial were limited to a gestational age of ≥32 weeks, ≤30 days of age, and ≥1800 g at the initiation of therapy, which decreased in part the generalizability of the conclusion.

Other Relevant Studies and Information:
- Subsequent to the publication of VGCV, oral valganciclovir for 6 months was accepted as a treatment option in the global recommendation for congenitally infected neonates with moderately to severely symptomatic CMV disease.[5,6]
- Bilavsky et al.[7] observed that in infants with symptomatic CMV infection who started antiviral treatment during the first 4 weeks of life and received this treatment for 12 months, hearing status was significantly improved. Even in cases of severe hearing loss at birth, 40% of ears benefited from antiviral treatment.
- There remains little evidence to guide treatment of more immature infants (<32 weeks' gestational age), those who are less symptomatic with congenital CMV, or those who remain untreated beyond 4 weeks of age.

Summary and Implications: The VGCV trail showed that 6 months of oral valganciclovir for symptomatic congenital CMV increases the likelihood of improved total hearing and neurodevelopmental outcomes at 24 months, without increasing the risk of adverse events. The results of this trial led to practice change in the treatment of infants with symptomatic CMV.

A CONVERSATION WITH THE TRIALIST: DAVID W. KIMBERLIN

Are there any new safer drugs that should be formally evaluated, such as the nontoxic, orally available agent, letermovir etc., before the CMV vaccine is available?

We are starting later this year a study of letermovir in neonates with symptomatic congenital CMV disease. This first study is a pharmacokinetic/pharmacodynamic investigation, but our hope is to follow this with a study of the combination of valganciclovir and letermovir initially followed by one of those drugs as monotherapy for the remainder of the treatment course. If we find letermovir to be effective on virologic control, I would be hopeful that it might be the one selected for the monotherapy portion of the treatment course to get away from the toxicities of valganciclovir.

Since there is no strong evidence in the management of mildly symptomatic or asymptomatic cytomegalovirus infection infants, what are your thoughts on how to do the decision-making when facing these specific infants?

This can be really challenging. I can say with certainty that neonates who are totally asymptomatic should not be treated. We recently stopped a study of valganciclovir in this population due to unacceptable toxicity: 43% developed Grade 3 or 4 neutropenia. The "mildly symptomatic" group is trickier, though, since there is not a strict definition of mild, moderate, and severe congenital CMV disease. I can say that our studies that showed benefit were in the type of baby who you could walk through the NICU and recognize had something wrong with them—small head, protuberant abdomen, petechiae, etc. I think this is the type of congenital CMV patient that should be considered for treatment. Additionally, we completed a placebo controlled trial of valganciclovir started beyond the first month of life and there was no benefit whatsoever, so when treatment is used in congenital CMV it must be initiated within the first month following delivery.

References

1. Kimberlin DW, Jester PM, Sanchez PJ, et al. Valganciclovir for symptomatic congenital cytomegalovirus disease. *N Engl J Med.* 2015;372:933–43.
2. Kimberlin DW, Lin C-Y, Sánchez PJ, et al. Effect of ganciclovir therapy on hearing in symptomatic congenital cytomegalovirus disease involving the central nervous system: a randomized, controlled trial. *J Peds.* 2003;143:16–25.
3. Pickering LK, Baker CJ, Long SS, et al. *Red Book: 2012 Report of the Committee on Infectious Diseases.* 29th ed. Elk Grove Village, IL: American Academy of Pediatrics; 2012. Cytomegalovirus infection:300–5.
4. Kimberlin DW, Acosta EP, Sánchez PJ, et al. Pharmacokinetic and pharmacodynamic assessment of oral valganciclovir in the treatment of symptomatic congenital cytomegalovirus disease. *J Infect Dis.* 2008; 197:836–45.
5. Rawlinson WD, Boppana SB, Fowler KB, et al. Congenital cytomegalovirus infection in pregnancy and the neonate: consensus recommendations for prevention, diagnosis, and therapy. *Lancet Infect Dis.* 2017 Jun;17(6):e177–e188.
6. Luck SE, Wieringa JW, Blázquez-Gamero D, et al. Congenital cytomegalovirus: a European expert consensus statement on diagnosis and management. *Pediatr Infect Dis J.* 2017;36(12):1205.
7. Bilavsky E, Shahar-Nissan K, Pardo J, et al. Hearing outcome of infants with congenital cytomegalovirus and hearing impairment. *Arch Dis Child.* 2016 May;101(5):433–8.

Hematology

29

Hemorrhagic Disease of the Newborn

Breastfeeding as a Necessary Factor in the Pathogenesis

ANNA E. CURLEY

"The present studies, reinforced by experience of the past, emphasize the efficacy and safety of small doses of vitamin K in the prevention of serious neonatal bleeding in the breast-fed infant who is at risk."
—SUTHERLAND ET AL.[1]

Research Question: Among newborn term infants, does prophylactic intramuscular (IM) vitamin K (100 µg or 5 mg), compared with 0.9% saline, decrease the frequency of hemorrhagic disease of the newborn (HDN) before hospital discharge?

Why Was This Study Done: At the time of this study, the American Academy of Pediatrics had recommended routine use of parenteral vitamin K (0.5 to 1 mg per dose) for all newborn infants,[2] which was based on observational data indicating benefit in mortality from bleeding.[3] However, the authors describe "vacillating practice: various preparations, various doses" and even "various opinions" about the need for any vitamin K.

Year Study Began: 1962

Year Study Published: 1967

Study Location: United States (single center)

Who Was Studied: Term infants weighing ≥2.26 kg (5 lbs) admitted to the newborn nursery.

Who Was Excluded: Exclusion criteria were not specified.

How Many Patients: 3,338

Study Overview: This study was a multi-arm, masked RCT (Figure 29.1).

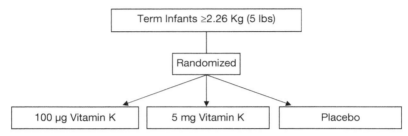

Figure 29.1 Study Overview

What Were the Interventions:
- Infants randomized vitamin K received their respective doses of menadione sodium bisulfite (synthetic preparation of vitamin K).
- Infants randomized to placebo received 0.9% normal saline.

All study interventions were given in a 0.5 mL volume administered intramuscularly on admission to the "full-term" stable newborn nursery.

How Long Was Follow-up: Hospital discharge which typically occurred at 84 to 110 hours of age, post-natal ages 4 to 5 days.

What Were the Endpoints:
Primary outcome: Clinical bleeding; subdivided by severity as severe (occurring in a significant location [central nervous system or adrenal] or associated with anemia or hypovolemia), moderate (occurring at innocuous sites and requiring local hemostatic measures), or minor (occurring at innocuous sites and not requiring hemostasis).
Secondary outcomes: Hyperbilirubinemia (>15 mg/100 mL), markers of coagulation in bleeding infants.

Concerns Regarding Bias: Although a similar volume was administered to all treatment arms, the study was at potential risk for performance bias, as vitamin K preparations compared with saline may have a different color, allowing differentiation between placebo and vitamin K groups. It is possible that some additional bias in the assessment of both efficacy and possible side effects (hyperbilirubinemia) existed, as not every infant was specifically examined. This was ameliorated by ensuring all ward personnel recorded any bleeds; and likely would not affect severe or moderately severe category of bleed coming to clinical attention.

RESULTS

- The incidence of any bleeding was 7.5% in the placebo group compared with 5.3% in the 100 µg vitamin K group and 5.7% in the 5 mg vitamin K group (p <0.025).
- Fewer infants who received any vitamin K had moderate/severe bleeding (0.3 to 0.4% versus 1.7%; p <0.0005).
- Severe bleeding occurred only in the placebo group, at a rate of 1:150 infants (p <0.0005).
- There was twice as much bleeding among the breastfed infants who received no vitamin K, compared with infants who received vitamin K or cow's milk formula or both.

Criticisms and Limitations: The investigators chose to trial a much smaller dose (100 µg) and much larger dose of Vitamin K3 or menadione than that suggested by the AAP at the time.[2] This may have been because of reported concerns about hyperbilirubinemia. Although the investigators reported hyperbilirubinemia >15 mg/dL, it is not clear that this was a prespecified outcome, and collection of data appeared to be pragmatic ("values in excess of 15 mg/100 mL are seldom overlooked").

Minor bleeding was not well reported; there were only 4 infants with cephalohematoma, 1 with ecchymosis, and 2 with petechiae reported in 3,338 infants. This is unlikely to have been a significant problem, however, as moderate and severe bleeding were more relevant outcomes.

The trial monitored bleeding to discharge (usually day 4 to 5) and would have potentially missed episodes of classic HDN (now referred to as vitamin K deficiency bleeding, VKDB) up to day 7. The authors sought to differentiate HDN from other causes of hemorrhage through an initial prothombin test. However, coagulation tests were not performed in 34% of bleeding infants.

Of note, the drug formulation used in this study was menadione sodium bisulfite (vitamin K3) which is a synthetic, water-soluble vitamin. This formulation is no longer in use as prophylaxis for VKDB because of its potential to cause hemolytic anemia and jaundice.

Other Relevant Studies and Information:
- In 1943, Dam and Doisy were awarded the Nobel Prize for their work on identifying and isolating vitamin K.[4]
- Despite strong recommendations for the past 6 decades, parent refusal of prophylactic vitamin K represents a growing trend, in part due to unfounded concerns for childhood cancer or fear of unnecessary discomfort for their infants. While the option for an oral formulation may be appealing, this treatment has not demonstrated sufficient efficacy in late-onset VKDB.[5] Early home discharge in modern neonatology makes refusal of prophylaxis a further concern.

Summary and Implications: This large RCT demonstrated that vitamin K prophylaxis effectively reduces HDN. It also demonstrated that lower doses of vitamin K were effective in preventing bleeding and identified breastfeeding as a major risk factor for hemorrhage, with a resultant 15 to 20-fold increase in moderate and severe bleeding without vitamin K. The trial aided in widespread acceptance of vitamin K as a standard treatment for all newborn infants.

A FEW WORDS FROM THE EDITOR

Before there was COVID immunization to divide parents and caregivers, there was vitamin K.

Sutherland and colleagues clearly demonstrated decreased bleeding in breastfed infants receiving intramuscular vitamin K. Despite this compelling evidence, the frequency of refusal of intramuscular vitamin K by parents ranges from 0% to 3.2% in US hospitals to a fourfold increase in refusal in the setting of home births.[1] Reasons for hesitancy include concerns for harms from the injection, a desire to be "natural," and a belief that there may be alternatives to vitamin K prophylaxis, including changes in maternal diet. Parents who decline intramuscular vitamin K tend to decline other preventive measures, including the hepatitis B vaccine at birth, prophylaxis against gonococcal ophthalmia, and subsequent routine vaccinations. Many parents and caregivers hope to substitute oral vitamin K, as an approach that avoids intramuscular injection but ignores the many epidemiological studies that show increased risk of late VKDB.[2] How to talk to parents? Caregivers need to be well versed in the important effects of vitamin K prophylaxis and an understanding of the perceived barriers.

—Roger Soll

1. Loyal J, Shapiro ED. Refusal of intramuscular vitamin K by parents of newborns: a review. *Hosp Pediatr.* 2020;10(3):286–94.
2. Levin R, Jung JM, Forrey L, et al. Refusal of vitamin K injection: survey of the current literature and practical tips for pediatricians. *Pediatr Ann.* 2018;47(8):e334–e338.

References

1. Sutherland JM, Glueck HI, Gleser G. Hemorrhagic disease of the newborn. Breast feeding as a necessary factor in the pathogenesis. *Am J Dis Child.* 1967;113(5):524–33.
2. American Academy of Pediatrics, Report of Committee on Nutrition: vitamin K compounds and the water-soluble analogues: use in therapy and prophylaxis in pediatrics. *Pediatrics.* 1961;28:501–7.
3. Lehmann J. Vitamin K as a prophylactic in 13,000 infants. *Lancet.* 1944;243:493–94.
4. Raju TN. The Nobel chronicles. 1943: Henrik Carl Peter Dam (1895–1976); and Edward Adelbert Doisy (1893–1986). *Lancet.* 1999;353(9154):761.
5. Hand I, Noble L, Abrams SA; Committee on Fetus and Newborn, Section on Breastfeeding, Committee on Nutrition. Vitamin K and the newborn infant. *Pediatrics.* March 2022;149(3):e2021056036.

30

Effects of Early Erythropoietin Therapy on the Transfusion Requirements of Preterm Infants Below 1250 Grams Birth Weight

ANNA E. CURLEY

"When conservative transfusion guidelines are followed, the combination of erythropoietin and iron as used in this trial does not have a significant impact on the number of transfusions administered to very low birth weight infants."

—OHLS ET AL.[1]

Research Question: Among very to extremely low birth weight preterm infants, does erythropoietin (EPO), as compared with placebo, decrease transfusion requirements?

Why Was This Study Done: Prior to this trial there had been several trials examining the role of EPO in preventing or treating anemia, thereby reducing or eliminating red cell transfusion in preterm infants. These studies were small, had less restrictive transfusion policies, and varied in timing of administration of EPO. Their findings suggested that EPO administration in preterm babies helped prevent transfusion,[2,3] but larger studies were required.

Year Study Began: Not stated

Year Study Published: 2001

Study Location: United States (8 centers)

Who Was Studied: Infants ≥401 g and ≤1250 g birth weight.

Who Was Excluded: Infants with a major congenital anomaly, a positive direct antiglobulin test, evidence of coagulopathy, clinical seizures, systolic blood pressure >100 mm Hg (in the absence of pressor support), or an absolute neutrophil count of ≤500/microliter.

How Many Patients:

Trial 1: 172 patients (90% power for a sample size of 160, to detect a minimum reduction from an anticipated 8 to 4 transfusions).

Trial 2: 118. Of note, the study had 90% power for a sample size of 200, to detect a decrease in the percentage of infants who received any transfusion from an anticipated 75% to 50%.

Study Overview: This study was comprised of 2 parallel-group, masked RCTs (Figure 30.1).

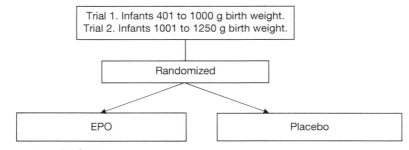

Figure 30.1 Study Overview

What Were the Interventions:
- Infants randomized to the intervention group received EPO 400 U/kg 3 times weekly as an intravenous infusion (IV) or subcutaneously.
- Infants in the placebo group received IV placebo or sham subcutaneous injections.

All study interventions were administered from between 24 and 96 hours of life to 35 weeks' PMA. All infants received supplemental parenteral and enteral iron, folate, and vitamin E. Strict transfusion criteria were followed based on hematocrit or hemoglobin levels and level of respiratory support.

How Long Was Follow-up: Hospital discharge or 120 days, whichever came first.

What Were the Endpoints:
Primary outcome: Number of transfusions per infant (Trial 1); percentage of babies transfused (Trial 2).
Selected secondary outcomes: Common complications of prematurity (including BPD, NEC, and late onset sepsis), mortality, absolute reticulocyte counts.

Concerns Regarding Bias: Absolute reticulocyte counts were significantly higher in the treatment group throughout the study in both trials ($p <0.001$), which could have partially unmasked the treatment group. Additional bias may be present with early termination of study enrollment in Trial 2.

RESULTS

Trial 1
- No difference in the number of transfusions received by each infant was detected with EPO (4.3 [standard deviation 3.6] versus 5.2 [4.2]; $p = 0.09$)
- No difference in transfusions during the study period was noted (84% versus 87%; $p = 0.56$), nor in total volume per infant who received a transfusion (80 [53] versus 95 [63] mL/kg; $p = 0.16$).

Trial 2
- There was no difference in the percentage of infants who received any transfusion with EPO (37% versus 46%; $p = 0.25$).
- No difference in the number of transfusions received by each infant was detected (1.0 [1.6] versus 1.1 [1.5]; $p = 0.42$).

There were no significant differences in morbidities or mortality in either trial.

Criticisms and Limitations: The 2 trials were designed to achieve a meaningful clinical difference that would be sufficient to warrant using a relatively intensive therapy by injection. The authors' anticipated effect size for these clinical differences were large.

Although the trial achieved similar baseline characteristics (including similar phlebotomy losses prior to enrollment), the phlebotomy losses in all babies

<1000 g at birth were high (on average approximately 100 mL/kg phlebotomy losses from birth in treatment and control groups). It would have been challenging for any drug to generate enough erythropoiesis to counteract this degree of iatrogenic anemia and prevent the necessity for transfusion. Of note, the investigators did see a reduction in the need for transfusion beyond week 7, consistent with the physiologically delayed onset of EPO effect and natural reduction in phlebotomy losses in babies at a median gestational age of 33 weeks. It is hard to judge what the effect of EPO might be 2 decades after this trial was completed, with the advent of delayed cord clamping and reduced phlebotomy losses through increased use of point of care testing.

The authors were careful to use a clear and restrictive transfusion policy across centers.

Although there was good compliance with the transfusion protocol in trial 1 (13% overall, compared with a predicted 10%), trial 2 showed less compliance (29% noncompliance in the EPO group versus 17%; $p = 0.14$).

Trial 2 was terminated early following randomization of 118 of 200 planned patients. This followed closure of trial 1 and interim review of the data by the Data and Safety Monitoring Committee, which suggested that trial 2 would be unlikely to demonstrate effectiveness of EPO in achieving the primary outcome. As a result, the ability to draw definitive conclusions from this trial is limited.

Other Relevant Studies and Information:
- A recent Cochrane meta-analysis of 34 studies, enrolling 3643 infants, compared erythropoiesis-stimulating agents in preterm or low birth weight infants versus a control consisting of placebo or no treatment and found that early EPO reduced the risk of "use of one or more red cell transfusions."[4] They estimated, however, that the total reduction in volume of red cells transfused per infant was small. The number of red cell transfusions per infant was also minimally reduced, and donor exposure was unchanged.
- Follow-up data from the Trial 1 cohort demonstrated similar growth, rehospitalization rates, and neurodevelopmental outcomes at 18 to 22 months' CA.[5]
- Meta-analysis of EPO (including the Trial 1 follow-up data) reported potential improvements in neurodevelopment.[4] However, subsequent larger trial investigation of higher doses of early EPO for potential neuroprotective effect showed no significant effect on death or severe neurodevelopmental impairment (See PENUT, Chapter 32).

Summary and Implications: This trial aimed to optimize patient selection, dose of EPO (although this was not varied), nutritional supplementation, and timing of therapy (early <96 hours) in combination with more restrictive guidelines in order to achieve a clinically meaningful reduction in red cell transfusion in preterm infants. Despite successfully inducing erythropoiesis, with significantly elevated reticulocyte counts, EPO did not significantly reduce transfusion requirements. Current review of evidence from RCTs of early EPO does not support its use in preterm infants.

A CONVERSATION WITH THE TRIALIST: ROBIN OHLS

What, if any, do you believe are the indications for EPO today, and are further trials needed to delineate these?

For infants less than 1250 grams, we start Darbe [darbepoetin] in the first week of life. . . . I don't think further placebo-controlled trials are needed to confirm the use of Epo or Darbe to stimulate red cell growth and increase red cell mass. We are currently performing a pilot study comparing once weekly dosing with every other week dosing (a more common dosing schedule in adults).

The use of Epo or Darbe to improve neurodevelopmental outcomes continues to be evaluated. We reported an improvement in our smaller multicenter study, but could not replicate it in the most recently completed NRN [Neonatal Research Network] study. . . . The mechanism for potential neurodevelopmental improvements is three-fold: 1) possible direct biologic effects of Epo or Darbe on neuronal progenitors and oligodendrocytes (the big unknown in humans), 2) increased hematocrit, and 3) decreased transfusions. We are still analyzing our data from our most recent Darbe trial performed in the NRN.

Can you tell us more about the thought process behind determining the parameters for a clinically meaningful effect in this study?

For the first Epo study performed in the NRN, we hypothesized that Epo would decrease transfusions in <1000 gram infants and increase the percent of 1001–1250 gram infants who remained un-transfused. I think we downplayed the results (and should have used Poisson regression instead of repeated measures) because there was a statistical decrease by week 7 of the study. Multiple studies since that first trial have proven that Epo and Darbe significantly decrease transfusion need. The argument that Epo and Darbe do not completely eliminate all transfusions is a bit disingenuous—you could say the same for surfactant or therapeutic hypothermia, yet the use of these treatments is embedded in NICU clinical care.

References

1. Ohls RK, Ehrenkranz RA, Wright LL, et al. Effects of early erythropoietin therapy on the transfusion requirements of preterm infants below 1250 grams birth weight: a multicenter, randomized, controlled trial. *Pediatrics*. 2001;108(4):934–42.
2. Ohls RK, Harcum J, Schibler KR, et al. The effect of erythropoietin on the transfusion requirements of preterm infants weighing 750 grams or less: a randomized, double-blind, placebo-controlled study. *J Pediatr*. 1997;131(5):661–5.
3. Brown MS, Keith JF 3rd. Comparison between two and five doses a week of recombinant human erythropoietin for anemia of prematurity: a randomized trial. *Pediatrics*. 1999 Aug;104(2 Pt 1):210–5.
4. Ohlsson A, Aher SM. Early erythropoiesis-stimulating agents in preterm or low birth weight infants. *Cochrane Database Syst Rev*. 2020;2(2):CD004863.
5. Ohls RK, Ehrenkranz RA, Das A, et al. Neurodevelopmental outcome and growth at 18 to 22 months' corrected age in extremely low birth weight infants treated with early erythropoietin and iron. *Pediatrics*. 2004;114(5):1287–91.

Higher or Lower Hemoglobin Transfusion Thresholds for Preterm Infants

The TOP Trial

AXEL R. FRANZ

"A higher hemoglobin threshold for transfusion was associated with an increased number of transfusions administered. However, it did not improve survival without impairment at 22 to 26 months of age. . . ."
—KIRPALANI ET AL.[1]

Research Question: In preterm infants with a gestational age <29 weeks, do higher hemoglobin thresholds for red-cell transfusions, as compared with lower thresholds, reduce the incidence of death or neurodevelopmental impairment (NDI) at 22 to 26 months' CA?

Why Was This Study Done: Extremely preterm infants universally develop anemia of prematurity. The capacity of compensatory mechanisms in response to anemia may be limited in preterm infants, and oxygen delivery in anemic infants may be particularly impaired during intermittent hypoxemic episodes, which are not only very common in very preterm infants but also associated with impaired neurodevelopmental outcome.[2]

Year Study Began: 2012

Year Study Published: 2020

Study Location: United States (19 centers, 41 NICUs)

Who Was Studied: Infants with a birth weight ≤1000 g, a gestational age between 22 and 28 weeks, and a postnatal age ≤48 hours.

Who Was Excluded: Infants considered to be nonviable, with major anomalies, or with suspicion for a blood anomaly based on family or prenatal history. Additionally, infants who received a prior red-cell transfusion after 6 hours of life were excluded.

How Many Patients: 1824

Study Overview: The TOP (Transfusion of Prematures) trial was a parallel-group, unmasked RCT (Figure 31.1).

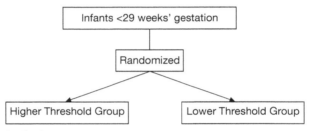

Figure 31.1 Study Overview

What Were the Interventions:
From randomization to 36 weeks' PMA, routine erythrocyte transfusions were guided by transfusion trigger algorithms taking into account postnatal age and respiratory support (e.g., high hemoglobin thresholds of 13 g/dL [8.07 mmol/L] for critically ill infants during the first week of life and 10 g/dL [6.21 mmol/L] for older, stable infants; low hemoglobin thresholds for similar infants were 11 g/dL [6.83 mmol/L] and 7 g/dL [4.34 mmol/L], respectively.). The goal difference in the pretransfusion hemoglobin levels was 2.0 to 2.5 g/dL [1.24 to 1.55 mmol/L] between treatment groups.

How Long Was Follow-up: 22 to 26 months' CA

What Were the Endpoints:
Primary outcome: Composite outcome of death or NDI.

Selected secondary outcomes: Death; individual components considered for NDI (cognitive delay, moderate to severe cerebral palsy, severe vision or hearing loss); severe complications of prematurity including NEC.

Concerns Regarding Bias: The study was at high risk for performance/detection bias, as caregivers were not blinded to the intervention. However, death is a robust/objective outcome, and assessors of neurodevelopment were blinded to treatment group assignment.

RESULTS

- No difference in the composite primary outcome of death or NDI was detected between the higher threshold group (50.1%) and the lower threshold group (49.8%) at 22 to 26 months CA (adjusted relative risk (aRR) 1.00, 95% CI 0.92 to 1.10, $p = 0.93$).
- No differences in the components of the primary outcome were detected between the treatment groups (death 16.2% versus 15.0%; aRR 1.07, 95% CI 0.87 to 1.32; and NDI 39.6% versus 40.3%; aRR 1.00, 95% CI 0.88 to 1.13) at 22–26 months' CA.
- No difference was detected in the rates of any of the common complications of prematurity, including NEC.

Criticisms and Limitations: The TOP trial was a pragmatic trial with several inherent limitations. The most important of these is that blinding of caregivers and parents was not possible, although outcome assessors were blinded. Additionally, this trial required prior transfusion algorithms be set aside temporarily. Lack of equipoise around lower-range hemoglobin levels likely contributed to the larger proportion of transfusions outside of study parameters in this group. Nonetheless, these were infrequent (3.5% of all red-cell transfusions), and near-target mean hemoglobin difference was achieved between the groups. Finally, blood bank practices varied by center; but randomization was stratified by center, and analyses aimed to adjust for center differences. Overall, the trial's pragmatic approach, with allowance for usual clinical variation, should enhance the generalizability of the study findings.

Future trials may consider assessing more individualized approaches to blood transfusion considering markers of tissue hypoxia instead of hemoglobin or hematocrit thresholds.

One concern may be that 2-year follow-up is insufficient to assess more subtle effects on longer-term cognitive or behavioral development, including, for example, executive functions, autism spectrum, or attention deficit disorders. The good news is that a longer-term follow-up study of the TOP cohort is underway (NCT01702805).

Other Relevant Studies and Information:
- Prior to this study, the largest trial on higher versus lower transfusion thresholds published before 2012, the PINT (Premature Infants in Need of Transfusion) trial,[3,4] which had involved more than 450 infants, indicated on post hoc analyses that there may be a reduced risk of mild-moderate cognitive delay with higher hemoglobin trigger thresholds. These results informed the design of the TOP trial as well as the design of the ETTNO (Effects of Transfusion Thresholds on Neurocognitive Outcome) trial.[5]
- Transfusion thresholds applied in TOP were consistent with those in common practice based on an international survey.[6]
- The ETTNO trial was conducted in 31 NICUs in Europe, and recruited 1013 infants with birth weights <1000 g, with randomization to very similar hematocrit transfusion triggers.[5] The results of ETTNO were strikingly similar to those of TOP: there was no difference in the primary outcome of death or NDI at 24±2 months CA (44.4% versus 42.9%), and there were no differences in the rates of the components of the primary outcome nor for common complications of prematurity including NEC. Despite similar transfusion triggers, the number of transfusions and total volume transfused was much lower in ETTNO than in TOP.

Summary and Implications: The TOP trial convincingly showed that higher transfusion triggers do not improve the rate of death or NDI at 22 to 26 months' CA. No other beneficial or harmful effects of higher transfusions triggers were found. Adoption of lower hemoglobin thresholds as used in TOP should reduce transfusions and transfusion-associated risks, while achieving similar outcomes at 2 years' CA.

A CONVERSATION WITH THE TRIALIST: HARESH KIRPALANI

How confident can we be about the results of the TOP trial?
In general, we gauge our confidence in trial results by how broad the CI around the mean of effect measures were; the internal validity of the trial; and whether

there has been replication. I think on all 3 grounds—including the replication by ETTNO—we can be reasonably confident about these results. Internal validity may be questioned by the non-adherence to algorithm violations; however this was in the end only a small number—and for ethical and pragmatic reasons, this could not have been designed differently in my view.

Is there a particularly high-risk subpopulation for which you would feel that the restrictive transfusion practice is perhaps not meeting their needs?

I do not think so if we are only talking about subgroups by weight or gestational age. If, however, we are considering specific patho-physiological states, we might have to pause. After all, TOP only examined stable but "anaemic" infants. In such instances it is possible that the oxygen supply–demand curves are different enough to warrant further trials. For instance, infants undergoing surgical procedures; or florid ductal opening, or equivalent steal or heart failures diagnoses.

References

1. Kirpalani H, Bell EF, Hintz SR, et al. Higher or lower hemoglobin transfusion thresholds for preterm infants. *N Engl J Med.* 2020;383(27):2639–51.
2. Poets CF, Roberts RS, Schmidt B, et al. Association between intermittent hypoxemia or bradycardia and late death or disability in extremely preterm infants. *JAMA.* 2015;314(6):595–603.
3. Kirpalani H, Whyte RK, Andersen C, et al. The Premature Infants in Need of Transfusion (PINT) study: a randomized, controlled trial of a restrictive (low) versus liberal (high) transfusion threshold for extremely low birth weight infants. *J Pediatr.* 2006;149(3):301–7.
4. Whyte RK, Kirpalani H, Asztalos EV, et al. Neurodevelopmental outcome of extremely low birth weight infants randomly assigned to restrictive or liberal hemoglobin thresholds for blood transfusion. *Pediatrics.* 2009;123(1):207–13.
5. Franz AR, Engel C, Bassler D, et al. Effects of liberal vs restrictive transfusion thresholds on survival and neurocognitive outcomes in extremely low-birth-weight infants: the ETTNO Randomized Clinical Trial. *JAMA.* 2020;324(6):560–70.
6. Guillen U, Cummings JJ, Bell EF, et al. International survey of transfusion practices for extremely premature infants. *Semin Perinatol.* 2012;36(4):244–7.

32

A Randomized Trial of Erythropoietin for Neuroprotection in Preterm Infants

The PENUT Trial

NICHOLAS D. EMBLETON

> "We did not observe that treatment with high-dose erythropoietin in extremely preterm infants resulted in a lower risk of death or better neurodevelopmental outcomes at 2 years of age."
>
> —JUUL ET AL.[1]

Research Question: Does high-dose erythropoietin (EPO) reduce death or severe neurodevelopmental impairment (NDI) at 2 years in extremely preterm infants?

Why Was This Study Done: High-dose erythropoietin (EPO) was shown to have neuroprotective effects in preclinical studies.[2] Prior to this trial, meta-analysis of the few RCTs that reported on the effects of early EPO on neurodevelopment suggested potential benefit in preterm infants,[3] but clinical efficacy was uncertain.

Year Study Began: 2013

Year Study Published: 2020

Study Location: United States (19 centers)

Who Was Studied: Infants born between 24 and 27 weeks' gestation.

Who Was Excluded: Infants with life-threating anomalies, chromosomal anomalies, disseminated intravascular coagulation, twin-to-twin transfusion, hematocrit level >65%, hydrops fetalis, or known congenital infection.

How Many Patients: 941 infants were enrolled, of whom 741 underwent evaluation of efficacy at 2 years. Of note, this is slightly below the goal of 752 infants to achieve >80% power for a 25% relative risk reduction in NDI.

Study Overview: PENUT was a parallel-group, masked RCT (Figure 32.1).

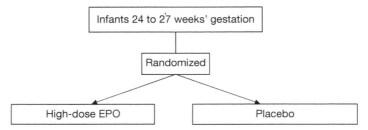

Figure 32.1 Study Overview

What Were the Interventions:
- Infants randomized to high-dose EPO received 1000 units/kg EPO intravenously within 24 hours of birth, with subsequent doses every 48 hours for a total of 6 doses. Thereafter, infants received maintenance subcutaneous injections of EPO at 400 units/kg 3 times per week until >32 weeks' PMA.
- Infants randomized to placebo received identical administrations of saline.

How Long Was Follow-up: 2 years' CA

What Were the Endpoints:
Primary outcome: Death or severe NDI at 22 to 26 months' PMA. Severe NDI was defined as composite motor or cognitive score <70 on the Bayley Scales of Infant and Toddler Development, Third Edition (BSID-III) or cerebral palsy (Gross Motor Function Classification Score, GMFCS, >2 out of 5).

Selected secondary outcomes: Death or moderate-to-severe NDI (GMFCS of 2, or BSID-III composite <85), separate components of the primary outcome, adverse events, and common neonatal morbidities.

Concerns Regarding Bias: This study was at risk of bias through its high attrition rate. This compounded the power problem noted above, with only 80% in each arm of enrolled infants available for "per-protocol efficacy analysis."

RESULTS

- Death or severe NDI occurred in 26% children in both groups (RR 1.03; 95% CI 0.81 to 1.32, $p = 0.80$).
- Multiple imputation for missing data did not change the results.
- There was no difference in mortality, moderate NDI, serious adverse events, or common complications of prematurity.

Criticisms and Limitations: While there was a wealth of evidence regarding the use of EPO in the prevention and treatment of anemia of prematurity (See Chapter 30), less evidence was available on the impact of EPO on developmental outcomes. The PENUT trial used a higher dose of EPO than many previous studies, and was specifically powered to evaluate NDI. The intervention continued until 32 weeks' PMA based on the maximum period of oligodendrocyte vulnerability.[4] Based on this, with the trial providing a robust dose given over a critical time period, the negative outcomes are unlikely due to insufficient drug exposure.

Neurodevelopmental testing at 2 years of age is typical in neonatal RCTs. However, as discussed elsewhere, BSID III may lack the precision compared with more detailed cognitive assessment later in childhood.

Although earlier smaller trials suggested improvement in NDI, the PENUT trial failed to provide evidence of this phenomenon. The failure to demonstrate the anticipated improvements is consistent with the paradigm of repetition of studies with larger sample sizes often resulting in less impressive findings.[5]

Other Relevant Studies and Information:
- These results are inconsistent with conclusions of previous meta-analysis regarding reduction in NDI. Given the power and careful methodology of the PENUT trial, its conclusion is more likely to be reliable.

- Previous concerns of a higher rate of ROP in EPO-treated infants[3] were not shown in this trial, and no other safety concerns were raised.
- Consistent with previous meta-analysis, post hoc analyses of the PENUT trial showed that the EPO dose used resulted in a lower number and volume of transfusions, and a lower rate of exposure to blood donors.[6]

Summary and Implications: This study strongly suggests that EPO does not result in fewer deaths or fewer cases of severe NDI, in contradiction to previously held beliefs. The study highlights the challenges of basing clinical practice on the results of a meta-analysis of a small number of underpowered RCTs.

A CONVERSATION WITH THE TRIALIST: SUNNY JUUL

Given the support from animal models and other smaller trials, do you think that there are other important studies to be done on EPO for neuroprotection, despite the results of the PENUT trial?

There are many questions remaining regarding Epo neuroprotection. At this point in our knowledge, it seems unlikely that any one drug will be the "silver bullet," and so the search is on for compatible, synergistic treatments.... We plan to evaluate several potential therapies alone and together to determine promising combinations.... I think it is work like this that will continue to move our field forward. Careful, reproducible work in multiple animal models will hopefully point the way to new therapeutic approaches.

Epo consistently is neuroprotective in many models, but incompletely, so it is possible that it can be used in conjunction with other neuroprotective agents to improve outcome. It may also be applicable as a monotherapy for term HIE. Studies are ongoing to determine this.

What would you say about improving attrition rates at 2-year outcomes for RCTs—how can we do better here?

Missing data from attrition rates is a huge problem and really can affect outcomes. This is particularly true because attrition is generally not random. Similarly, I think it is really important to include a diverse population when enrolling patients into a study so it will be generalizable. I don't have any great solutions, except perhaps to increase funding for the follow-up portion of studies. Funds for transportation, or for home visits for evaluations. Studies that have done this have better follow-up rates.

References

1. Juul SE, Comstock BA, Wadhawan R, et al.; PENUT Trial Consortium. A randomized trial of erythropoietin for neuroprotection in preterm infants. *N Engl J Med*. 2020;382(3): 233–43.
2. Rangarajan V, Juul SE. Erythropoietin: emerging role of erythropoietin in neonatal neuroprotection. *Pediatr Neurol*. 2014;51:481–8.
3. Ohlsson A, Aher SM. Early erythropoiesis-stimulating agents in preterm or low birth weight infants. *Cochrane Database Syst Rev*. 2017;11:CD004863.
4. Juul SE, Mayock DE, Comstock BA, et al. Neuroprotective potential of erythropoietin in neonates: design of a randomized trial. *Matern Health Neonatol Perinatol*. 2015;1:27.
5. Ioannidis JPA. Why most published research findings are false. *JAMA*. 2005;2(8):e124.
6. Juul SE, Vu PT, Comstock BA, et al.; Preterm Erythropoietin Neuroprotection Trial Consortium. Effect of high-dose erythropoietin on blood transfusions in extremely low gestational age neonates: post hoc analysis of a randomized clinical trial. *JAMA Pediatr*. 2020 Oct 1;174(10):933–43.

33

Effect of a Higher vs Lower Platelet Transfusion Threshold on Death or Major Bleeding in Preterm Infants

The PlaNeT-2 Trial

RAVI MANGAL PATEL

"This large, multicenter, randomized trial involving preterm infants with severe thrombocytopenia showed that more deaths, major bleeding, or both occurred when a higher prophylactic platelet-count transfusion threshold of 50,000 per cubic millimeter was used than when a threshold of 25,000 per cubic millimeter was used."

—CURLEY ET AL.[1]

Research Question: Among preterm infants <34 weeks' gestation with severe thrombocytopenia and no evidence of major hemorrhage, does a prophylactic platelet transfusion at a platelet count threshold of $50 \times 10^9/L$, as compared with $25 \times 10^9/L$, reduce the risk of death or major bleeding up to 28 days after randomization?

Why Was This Study Done: Prophylactic platelet transfusions at a platelet count threshold of $\geq 50 \times 10^9/L$ are common in neonates,[2] despite the lack of supporting RCT evidence evaluating clinically relevant outcomes.

Year Study Began: 2011

Year Study Published: 2019

Study Location: United Kingdom, Ireland, Netherlands (43 centers total)

Who Was Studied: Infants <34 weeks' gestation with severe thrombocytopenia, defined as a platelet count <50 × 10⁹/L, and no evidence of major IVH.

Who Was Excluded: Infants with major or life-threatening congenital malformation, major bleeding within 72 hours, fetal intracranial hemorrhage, immune thrombocytopenia, no administration of parenteral vitamin K, or a low probability of survival beyond several hours. Of note, infants with major bleeding could be eligible for randomization after 72 hours if there was no further major bleeding.

How Many Patients: 660

Study Overview: The PlaNeT-2 trial was a parallel-group, unmasked RCT (Figure 33.1).

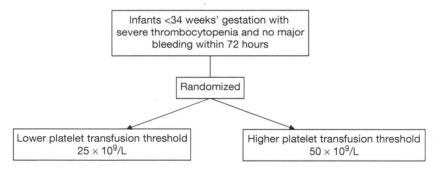

Figure 33.1 Study Overview

What Were the Interventions:
- Infants randomized to the lower platelet transfusion threshold received prophylactic platelet transfusion at a dose of 15 mL/kg when their platelet counts were <25 × 10⁹/L.
- Infants randomized to the higher platelet transfusion threshold received the same volume of transfusion when their platelet counts were <50 × 10⁹/L.

How Long Was Follow-up: 28 days post-randomization

What Were the Endpoints:
Primary outcome: Composite outcome of death or major bleeding, with bleeding prospectively assessed with a validated neonatal bleeding assessment tool.[3]
Selected secondary outcomes: Components of the primary outcome as well as grades of bleeding (minor, moderate, major), common complications of prematurity (including BPD), number of platelet-transfusion episodes, adverse events.

Concerns Regarding Bias: This study was at high risk for performance/detection bias or changes in co-treatments, as clinicians were not blinded to the intervention.

RESULTS

- Infants randomized to a higher platelet transfusion threshold had a higher risk of new major bleeding or death (26% versus 19%; adjusted odds ratio [OR] 1.57, 95% CI 1.06 to 2.32, $p = 0.02$).
- At least one platelet transfusion occurred in 90% of the infants in the higher threshold group, compared with 53% of infants in the lower threshold group (hazard ratio 2.75, 95% CI 2.36 to 3.21).
- Serious adverse events were not significantly different between higher and lower threshold groups.
- Infants randomized to the higher threshold group had a higher risk of survival with BPD (63% versus 54%; OR 1.54, 95% CI 1.03 to 2.30). There were no other differences in rates of common complications of prematurity.

Criticisms and Limitations: This is an important and well-conducted trial, although some potential limitations should be considered. The generalizability of the findings to very early transfusion thresholds may be limited, because 39% of the infants in the study had already received at least one platelet transfusion prior to randomization. It is possible that these transfusions occurred during the highest-risk period for bleeding in the first several days of life. However, subgroup analyses by postnatal age at randomization (<72 hours, 72 hours to <7 days, 7 days or more) did not show evidence of heterogeneity in effect estimates (interaction $p = 0.69$).

Interpretation of the study results may be further limited by varying etiologies of thrombocytopenia within the trial population. Infants with immune thrombocytopenia were excluded, but etiology was otherwise left largely unspecified, ultimately enrolling a patient population with a high background incidence of necrotizing enterocolitis and sepsis. Although these diagnoses may represent the majority of cases of thrombocytopenia seen in neonatal intensive care, it is unclear if infants with different causes for thrombocytopenia may respond differently at these transfusion thresholds.

The trial required a head ultrasound within 6 hours prior to randomization and excluded infants with significant IVH. It is understandable why this was done. However, in clinical practice, it may not always be possible to obtain a head ultrasound within that timeframe. Thus, clinical decisions regarding prophylactic platelet transfusion may be made without this information. It is unclear how this would impact the application of the trial findings in clinical settings without timely availability of cranial ultrasound.

Other Relevant Studies and Information:
- Prior to this trial, Andrew et al.[4] randomized 152 thrombocytopenic preterm infants during the first 72 hours of life to a platelet count transfusion threshold of 50 versus 150×10^9/L. The trial showed no difference between higher and lower thresholds in the primary outcome of new intracranial hemorrhage (28% versus 26%; $p = 0.73$).
- Although the Andrew et al. trial showed no benefit to a prophylactic platelet count transfusion threshold greater than 50×10^9/L, many preterm infants are routinely transfused at higher thresholds than this.[2]
- Platelet function (e.g., CT-ADP [closure time in response to adenosine diphosphate] assay) may be more important than platelet count in determining the risk of bleeding. One study showed a poor correlation between platelet count and bleeding score, which was contrasted by a stronger correlation between platelet function (measured using CT-ADP) and bleeding score.[5]
- The PlaNeT-2 cohort was followed for 2-year neurodevelopmental outcomes, with a higher rate of death or significant neurodevelopmental impairment observed in the higher platelet transfusion threshold group (50% versus 39%, $p = 0.017$).[6]

Summary and Implications: The PlaNeT-2 trial showed harm with the use of a prophylactic platelet count transfusion threshold of 50×10^9/L, compared with 25×10^9/L, for infants <34 weeks' gestation with severe thrombocytopenia. These findings support the use of a threshold of 25×10^9/L for prophylactic platelet transfusions. Importantly, the findings of this trial do not apply to neonates with major bleeding within the past 72 hours, where evidence is lacking to guide practice.

A CONVERSATION WITH THE TRIALIST: ANNA CURLEY

Do you think different etiologies for thrombocytopenia may respond differently to these transfusion thresholds?

Our study did not show a difference in babies with thrombocytopenia related to decreased production (intrauterine growth restriction) compared to those with an etiology likely related to both decreased synthesis and increased destruction (i.e., sepsis [415/660] and/or NEC [107/660]). Instead, I think that babies may be more likely to respond differently to thresholds, not related to etiology, but based on gestational age/severity of illness at the time of transfusion. Further analysis of our data ... suggested that smaller, sicker, more premature babies did even worse with higher transfusion thresholds.[1] Our study also showed a ... separation in primary outcome starting beyond the first week from platelet transfusion, suggesting that an inflammatory mechanism of harm might be, not just biologically, but also temporally plausible.

I would speculate that the worsened outcome in smaller sicker babies might be explained by their background increased inflammation in the lung and/or gut at the time of transfusion meaning that they were primed for greater harm.

What were the considerations in allowing recruitment of infants who had already received a platelet transfusion before randomization?

Recruiting these babies added a level of complexity to the study and its analysis, but on balance it also allowed for greater recruitment and prevented exclusion of a critically ill cohort. It allowed for a more representative sample of real life in neonatal intensive care. Most of the babies who had received transfusions prior to randomization were babies with a diagnosis of NEC who were transferred from lower acuity neonatal units to tertiary surgical units. It is possible that the background incidence of mortality/major bleed in a non-transfused population might have been lower and we might not have detected a real difference in outcome based on inadequate sample size if we had excluded pre-transfused babies. We also felt that randomization would allow for comparable numbers of pre-transfused babies in both threshold groups, and we were interested in the cumulative effect of platelet transfusions and overall platelet donor exposure rather than just a binary variable of 'transfused or not.'

1. Fustolo-Gunnink SF, Fijnvandraat K, van Klaveren D, et al. Preterm neonates benefit from low prophylactic platelet transfusion threshold despite varying risk of bleeding or death. *Blood.* 2019;134(26):2354–60.

References

1. Curley A, Stanworth SJ, Willoughby K, et al.; PlaNeT2 MATISSE Collaborators. Randomized trial of platelet-transfusion thresholds in neonates. *N Engl J Med.* 2019;380(3):242–51.
2. Patel RM, Hendrickson JE, Nellis ME, et al.; National Heart, Lung, and Blood Institute Recipient Epidemiology and Donor Evaluation Study-IV-Pediatric (REDS-IV-P). Variation in neonatal transfusion practice. *J Pediatr.* 2021;235:92–99.e4.
3. Venkatesh V, Curley A, Khan R, et al. A novel approach to standardised recording of bleeding in a high risk neonatal population. *Arch Dis Child Fetal Neonatal Ed.* 2013;98:F260–F263.
4. Andrew M, Vegh P, Caco C, et al. A randomized, controlled trial of platelet transfusions in thrombocytopenic premature infants. *J Pediatr.* 1993 Aug;123(2):285–91.
5. Deschmann E, Saxonhouse MA, Feldman HA, et al. Association of bleeding scores and platelet transfusions with platelet counts and closure times in response to adenosine diphosphate (CT-ADPs) among preterm neonates with thrombocytopenia. *JAMA Netw Open.* 2020 Apr 1;3(4):e203394.
6. Moore CM, D'Amore A, Fustolo-Gunnink S, et al.; PlaNeT2 MATISSE. Two-year outcomes following a randomised platelet transfusion trial in preterm infants. *Arch Dis Child Fetal Neonatal Ed.* 2023;108(5):452–7. doi: 10.1136/archdischild-2022-324915.

Ophthalmology

34

Multicenter Trial of Cryotherapy for Retinopathy of Prematurity

The CRYO-ROP Trial

JAMES I. HAGADORN

"These data support the efficacy of cryotherapy in reducing by approximately one-half the risk of unfavorable retinal outcome from threshold ROP."
— CRYOTHERAPY FOR RETINOPATHY OF PREMATURITY COOPERATIVE GROUP[1]

Research Question: Does transscleral cryotherapy of the avascular retina, versus no treatment, reduce the risk of poor visual acuity, in infants with severe ("threshold") ROP and weighing <1251 g at birth?

Why Was This Study Done: At the time of this study, use of cryotherapy for severe ROP was increasing globally, but RCTs defining its safety and efficacy were lacking.

Year Study Began: 1986

Year Study Published: 1988

Study Location: United States (23 centers)

Who Was Studied: Infants weighing <1251 g at birth who developed severe ROP (at least 5 contiguous or 8 cumulative 30° sectors [clock hours] of stage 3 ROP in zone 1 or 2, in the presence of plus disease).

Who Was Excluded: Infants with a lethal congenital anomaly or a major congenital ocular anomaly affecting one or both eyes.

How Many Patients: This paper reports the outcomes of the 172 infants that could be evaluated at follow-up for the last of several preplanned interim analyses. It demonstrated improved outcome in the intervention group at 3-month follow-up and led to early termination of study enrollment. At that time, a total of 291 infants had been randomized, slightly short of the target cohort of 300.

Study Overview: The CRYO-ROP (CRYOtherapy for Retinopathy of Prematurity) trial was a parallel-group, unmasked RCT. Randomization was stratified by either one eye (if asymmetric disease present) or both eyes (if symmetric disease) meeting criteria (Figure 34.1).

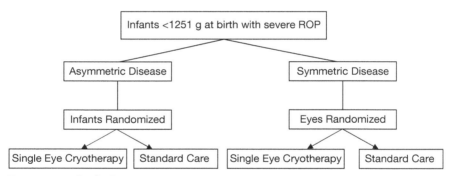

Figure 34.1 Study Overview

What Were the Interventions:
- Cryotherapy entailed transscleral cryotherapy of the avascular retina.
- Standard care entailed observation without intervention.

Randomization for infants with asymmetric disease was done on the infant level, whereas randomization for infants with symmetric disease was performed at the level of the eye.

Although not included in the analysis, infants with asymmetric disease who were randomized to standard care and went on to develop threshold disease in their less severely affected eye were offered cryotherapy for the second eye.

How Long Was Follow-up: 3 months post-treatment

What Were the Endpoints:
Primary outcome: Unfavorable structural outcome (defined as posterior retinal detachment, retinal fold involving the macula, or retrolental tissue that obscured the view of the posterior pole).
Secondary outcomes: Complications during cryotherapy.

Concerns Regarding Bias: The study was at high risk of performance/detection bias as personnel were not blinded to the intervention.

RESULTS

- At interim analysis, structural outcome was better at 3 months in eyes that received cryotherapy, as compared with untreated eyes (21.8% versus 43%; χ^2 20.5, p <0.0001).
- The most common complications during the procedure were hemorrhage (retinal, preretinal, or vitreous; 19.1%), conjunctival or subconjunctival hematoma (10.2%), and bradycardia or other arrhythmia (8.9%).

Criticisms and Limitations: The trial's unique design allowed all enrolled infants the opportunity to receive cryotherapy to one eye if threatened with the prospect of bilateral blindness. Similarly, the authors were reluctant to perform cryotherapy on both eyes because of potential long-term complications with the treatment. However, post-randomization treatments were not included in the analysis.

Four years after this publication, RCTs began reporting that laser photocoagulation produced comparable results.[2] Subsequent studies demonstrated that, compared with cryotherapy, laser was generally associated with lower rates of systemic complications (e.g., apnea, bradycardia, or arrhythmia), better structural outcomes, and less myopia and other adverse visual outcomes.[3] This "therapeutic instability" is typical of treatments in intensive care settings, where modifications or entirely new approaches quickly supplant proven therapy.

Other Relevant Studies and Information:
- Subsequent publications reported 3-month structural outcomes for the full randomized cohort,[4] structural and visual outcomes at 1 year,[5] 3.5 years,[6] 5.5 years,[7] 10 years,[8] and 15 years,[9] as well as a host of secondary analyses.

- Significant benefit from cryotherapy remained evident for structural and visual outcomes for 254 survivors through 15-year follow-up: 30% of treated and 51.9% of control eyes had unfavorable structural outcomes (p <0.001), while 44.7% of treated and 64.3% of control eyes had unfavorable visual acuity outcome (p <0.001).[9]
- Severe ROP meeting the "threshold" for enrollment in the CRYO-ROP randomized treatment cohort was defined using International Classification of ROP (ICROP) criteria[10] corresponding to retinal disease with an estimated 50% likelihood of progressing to blindness. The STOP-ROP trial[11] published in 2000 (See STOP-ROP, Chapter 35.) and ET ROP trial[12] in 2003 further refined this definition, resulting in recommendations for treatment of ROP earlier in its progression.
- In a separate series of publications, the authors followed all untreated infants (including all screened infants with no ROP or ROP not meeting treatment criteria and all eyes meeting treatment criteria but not randomized to receive cryotherapy).[13,14] This helped define the natural history of the disease, improved understanding of its epidemiology, and provided a strong new evidence basis for systematic ROP screening.

Summary and Implications: Although transscleral cryotherapy was quickly supplanted by retinal laser photocoagulation as the preferred procedure for surgical treatment of severe disease, the CRYO-ROP trial remains a defining landmark in the monitoring and treatment of ROP. It was the first large multi-center trial to use the ICROP classification system to describe ROP severity, and it was the first to demonstrate a convincing beneficial therapy for severe ROP. Subsequent trials advancing our knowledge of ROP progression and treatment rest upon this sturdy foundation.

A CONVERSATION WITH THE TRIALIST: BETTY TUNG, THE RESEARCH MANAGER FOR CRYO-ROP AND MANY SUBSEQUENT ROP TRIALS.

This was a unique and groundbreaking collaboration between ophthalmologists and neonatologists; can you give us more insight into this collaboration?

At the time of CRYO-ROP, there was no gold standard treatment for ROP. The ICROP committee had published a new classification system for ROP including zones, stages, and plus disease in 1984. The CRYO-ROP study expanded on the

ICROP system and defined a hierarchy of "lowest zone, highest stage." A unique feature of the CRYO-ROP study was that each center had a neonatologist as a study investigator. Dr. William Silverman was even a member of the Data & Safety Monitoring Committee.

The cooperative group for CRYO-ROP was a model for multidimensional studies, evaluating aspects including long-term follow-up, natural history, and intervention. How did you manage all this?

We wanted to do things right. Even though the early study outcome was published within 2 years, the visual outcomes and developmental outcomes were felt to be so important that further follow-up was desired. Thus, further follow-up at 5, 10, and even 15 years were studied. As you might imagine, having people follow up after so long a time could be difficult to achieve. The efforts of the study coordinators [were] so important to contact patients and schedule visits for this long-term follow up.

References

1. Cryotherapy for Retinopathy of Prematurity Cooperative Group. Multicenter trial of cryotherapy for retinopathy of prematurity: preliminary results. *Arch Ophthalmol.* 1988;106:471–9.

    Cryotherapy for Retinopathy of Prematurity Cooperative Group. Multicenter trial of cryotherapy for retinopathy of prematurity: preliminary results. *Pediatrics.* 1988 May;81(5):697–706.
2. McNamara J, Tasman W, Vander J, et al. Diode laser photocoagulation for retinopathy of prematurity: preliminary results. *Arch Ophthalmol.* 1992;110:1714–6.
3. Simpson J, Melia M, Yang M, et al. Current role of cryotherapy in retinopathy of prematurity: a report by the American Academy of Ophthalmology. *Ophthalmology.* 2012;119:873–7.
4. Cryotherapy for Retinopathy of Prematurity Cooperative Group. Multicenter trial of cryotherapy for retinopathy of prematurity: three-month outcome. *Arch Ophthalmol.* 1990;108:195–204.
5. Cryotherapy for Retinopathy of Prematurity Cooperative Group. Multicenter trial of cryotherapy for retinopathy of prematurity. One-year outcome--structure and function. *Arch Ophthalmol.* 1990;108:1408–16.
6. Cryotherapy for Retinopathy of Prematurity Cooperative Group. Multicenter trial of cryotherapy for retinopathy of prematurity. 3 1/2-year outcome--structure and function. *Arch Ophthalmol.* 1993;111:339–44.
7. Cryotherapy for Retinopathy of Prematurity Cooperative Group. Multicenter trial of cryotherapy for retinopathy of prematurity. Snellen visual acuity and structural outcome at 5 1/2 years after randomization. *Arch Ophthalmol.* 1996;114:417–24.
8. Cryotherapy for Retinopathy of Prematurity Cooperative Group. Multicenter trial of cryotherapy for retinopathy of prematurity. Ophthalmological outcomes at 10 years. *Arch Ophthalmol.* 2001;119:1110–8.

9. Palmer E, Hardy R, Dobson V, et al.; Cryotherapy for Retinopathy of Prematurity Cooperative Group. 15-year outcomes following threshold retinopathy of prematurity: final results from the Multicenter Trial of Cryotherapy for Retinopathy of Prematurity. *Arch Ophthalmol.* 2005;123:311–8.

10. Committee for the Classification of Retinopathy of Prematurity. An international classification of retinopathy of prematurity. *Arch Ophthalmol.* 1984;102:1130–4.

11. The STOP ROP Multicenter Study Group. Supplemental Therapeutic Oxygen for Prethreshold Retinopathy Of Prematurity (STOP-ROP), a randomized, controlled trial. I: primary outcomes. *Pediatrics.* 2000;105:295–310.

12. Early Treatment for Retinopathy of Prematurity Cooperative Group. Revised indications for the treatment of retinopathy of prematurity: results of the Early Treatment for Retinopathy of Prematurity randomized trial. *Arch Ophthalmol.* 2003;121:1684–94.

13. Cryotherapy for Retinopathy of Prematurity Cooperative Group. The natural ocular outcome of premature birth and retinopathy. Status at 1 year. *Arch Ophthalmol.* 1994;112:903–12.

14. Cryotherapy for Retinopathy of Prematurity Cooperative Group. Multicenter trial of cryotherapy for retinopathy of prematurity: natural history ROP: ocular outcome at 5(1/2) years in premature infants with birth weights less than 1251 g. *Arch Ophthalmol.* 2002;120:595–9.

35

Supplemental Therapeutic Oxygen for Prethreshold Retinopathy of Prematurity

The STOP-ROP Trial

SOUVIK MITRA

"By this analysis, one could expect ~1 episode of pneumonia/[BPD] exacerbation for each case of peripheral ablative surgery that might be prevented."
—THE STOP-ROP STUDY GROUP[1]

Research Question: Among preterm infants with confirmed prethreshold ROP in at least one eye, does supplemental oxygen therapy to achieve SpO_2 target range of 96% to 99%, compared with conventional oxygenation to achieve a SpO_2 (pulse oximeter oxygen saturation) target of 89% to 94%, reduce progression to threshold ROP requiring peripheral ablative surgery?

Why Was This Study Done: ROP is a neovascular retinal disorder in preterm infants. Its progression may be exacerbated by hypoxic stimuli leading to release of angiogenic growth factors. A previous observational study demonstrated that moderate supplemental oxygen (target SpO_2 99% with PaO_2 ≤ 100 mm Hg) was associated with regression of prethreshold ROP.[2]

Year Study Began: 1994

Year Study Published: 2000

Study Location: United States (30 centers)

Who Was Studied: Preterm infants with prethreshold ROP in at least one eye.

Who Was Excluded: Infants with lethal anomalies or congenital anomalies of the eye. Infants with a median oxygen saturation >94% in room air were deemed ineligible.

How Many Patients: Of the planned sample size of 880 to detect a one-third reduction in progression to threshold ROP (10% absolute reduction), only 649 infants were enrolled, due to slow patient accrual.

Study Overview: This was a parallel-group, unmasked RCT. Randomization was stratified by center and by 2 levels of baseline ROP severity (Figure 35.1).

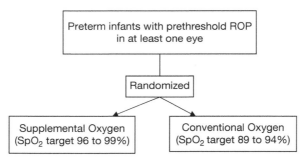

Figure 35.1 Study Overview

What Were the Interventions:
- Infants randomized to supplemental oxygen received supplemental oxygen titrated to maintain SpO_2 between 96% and 99%.
- Infants randomized to standard care received supplemental oxygen as needed to maintain SpO_2 between 89% and 94%.

All infants were placed on continuous pulse oximetry monitors set up to monitor, record, and report trends in oxygen saturation for each infant. After a minimum of 2 weeks, the assigned intervention was discontinued once both eyes reached primary ophthalmic outcomes.

How Long Was Follow-up: 3 months' CA

What Were the Endpoints:

Primary outcome: Progression of at least one eye to confirmed threshold ROP, determined by weekly eye examinations.

Selected secondary outcomes: Pneumonia and/or exacerbations of BPD, severe ophthalmic sequelae, prolonged hospitalization or re-hospitalization, prolonged need for supplemental oxygen therapy.

Concerns Regarding Bias: The study was at high risk for performance/ascertainment bias, as caregivers were not blinded to the intervention (Only outcome assessors were blinded.). In addition, the trial was stopped early; the Data and Safety Monitoring Board noted widening adoption of liberal, higher oxygen targeting in the community making patient accrual more difficult.

RESULTS

- The rate of progression to threshold ROP in at least one eye was 41% in the supplemental arm and 48% in the conventional arm. Adjusting for baseline ROP severity, plus disease, race, and gestational age; the odds ratio for ROP progression with supplemental oxygen was 0.72 (95% CI 0.52 to 1.01).
- Pneumonia and/or exacerbations of BPD were higher in the supplemental oxygen arm versus the conventional arm, although this did not reach statistical significance.
- At 3 months' CA, rates of severe ophthalmic sequelae were similar in both arms; rates of hospitalization and need for supplemental oxygen therapy were significantly higher in the supplemental oxygen arm.

Criticisms and Limitations: Two major issues common to RCTs present themselves in this trial. The first is the issue of what to do with an outcome that nears statistical significance, especially in a study closed early. Current GRADE (Grading of Recommendations Assessment, Development and Evaluation) recommendations[3] instruct us to pay close attention to the point estimate. For this trial, which demonstrates a 7% absolute reduction in progression to threshold ROP with supplemental oxygen with a confidence interval that approaches nominal statistical significance, one could plausibly conclude that the therapy *may* be effective for the primary outcome.

The second issue is what to do with apparently meaningful secondary outcomes and subgroup analyses. These outcomes may be unanticipated, as in the case of the 3-month pulmonary outcomes of this trial, and present the clinician with new concerns when approaching a therapy. Alternatively, the trial also reports a significant effect of supplemental oxygen on progression to threshold disease for the subgroup of infants without plus disease. Importantly, while definitive proof of effect would generally necessitate a prospective and adequately powered trial, these results of evolving evidence can impact subsequent research and NICU policy, making such a trial more difficult to achieve. The challenge for clinicians to balance this incomplete dataset remains, as the field awaits further evidence.

Other Relevant Studies and Information:
- A Cochrane review on "Supplemental oxygen for the treatment of prethreshold retinopathy of prematurity," last updated in 2003, identified the STOP-ROP trial as the only potentially eligible trial for this clinical question.[4] This highlights the dearth of RCT evidence in this area.

Summary and Implications: Despite a plausible biologic rationale, the STOP-ROP trial was unable to demonstrate a statistically significant reduction in progression of prethreshold ROP with higher target SpO_2 of 96% to 99%. The trial also suggested potential harm from higher target saturation goals, with more hospitalizations and adverse pulmonary outcomes at 3 months' CA. This important but underpowered trial describes potential trade-offs with higher oxygen saturation targets; however, the risks and benefits of targeting higher oxygen saturation in infants with prethreshold disease require further evaluation.

A FEW WORDS FROM THE EDITORS

The STOP-ROP trial presents the dilemma of achieving an appropriate balance with target oxygen saturations to optimize an infant's outcome. Do we need to individualize appropriate oxygenation saturation targets for each infant? At what age? What is the optimal outcome? A subgroup of patients in the STOP-ROP trial seemed to benefit from higher oxygen saturation goals. However, we are also confronted with an increase in pulmonary complications. Would families have a preference between avoiding ROP versus avoiding pulmonary sequelae? As our field continues to navigate into the unknown, efforts are increasing to include families and their distinct perspectives in this journey. For such therapies with likely trade-offs, the family vantage point as well as the individual infant's case should be considered.

—Susanne Hay & Roger Soll

References

1. The STOP-ROP Multicenter Study Group. Supplemental Therapeutic Oxygen for Prethreshold Retinopathy Of Prematurity (STOP-ROP), a randomized, controlled trial. I: primary outcomes. *Pediatrics*. 2000 Feb;105(2):295–310.
2. Gaynon MW, Stevenson DK, Sunshine P, et al. Supplemental oxygen may decrease progression of prethreshold disease to threshold retinopathy of prematurity. *J Perinatol*. 1997 Dec;17(6):434–8.
3. Santesso N, Glenton C, Dahm P, et al.; GRADE Working Group. GRADE guidelines 26: informative statements to communicate the findings of systematic reviews of interventions. *J Clin Epidemiol*. 2020;119:126–35.
4. Lloyd J, Askie L, Smith J, et al. Supplemental oxygen for the treatment of prethreshold retinopathy of prematurity. *Cochrane Database Syst Rev*. 2003;(2):CD003482.

36

Efficacy of Intravitreal Bevacizumab for Stage 3+ Retinopathy of Prematurity

The BEAT-ROP Trial

BRIAN CHRISTOPHER KING

"Intravitreal bevacizumab monotherapy, as compared with conventional laser therapy, in infants with stage 3+ retinopathy of prematurity showed a significant benefit for zone I but not zone II disease."
—MINTZ-HITTNER ET AL.[1]

Research Question: Does intravitreal bevacizumab monotherapy, compared with conventional laser therapy (standard of care), reduce the incidence of recurrent ROP among preterm infants with stage 3 ROP with plus disease (stage 3+ ROP) in zones I or II posterior through 54 weeks' postmenstrual age (PMA)?

Why Was This Study Done: At the time of this study, clinicians struggled with the treatment of zone I ROP, with a high incidence of recurrence after laser ablation.

Year Study Began: 2008

Year Study Published: 2011

Study Location: United States (15 centers)

Who Was Studied: Preterm infants born ≤30 weeks' gestation or with a birth weight ≤1500 grams were eligible for retinopathy screening. Infants with stage 3+ ROP in zone I or zone II posterior in each eye were eligible for enrollment.

Who Was Excluded: Infants with stage 4 or stage 5 ROP in either eye.

How Many Patients: 150.

Study Overview: The BEAT-ROP trial was a parallel group, unmasked, RCT (Figure 36.1); with randomization stratified by zone of disease (zone I or zone II posterior).

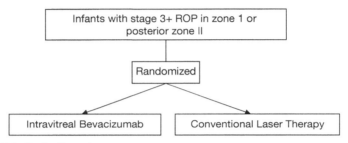

Figure 36.1 Study Overview

What Were the Interventions:
- Infants randomized to the intervention group received intravitreal bevacizumab, a vascular endothelial growth factor (VEGF) inhibitor, to both eyes.
- Infants randomized to the standard care group received conventional laser therapy to both eyes.

How Long Was Follow-up: One week and 1 month after any treatment, and at 54 weeks' PMA.

What Were the Endpoints:
Primary ocular outcome: Need for retreatment in either eye prior to 55 weeks' PMA.
    Selected secondary outcomes: Structural changes associated with unfavorable ocular outcomes (including dragging, distortion, or detachment of the macula).

Concerns Regarding Bias: The study was at high risk for performance/detection bias, as caregivers and evaluating ophthalmologists were not blinded to the intervention. There was also unclear risk of bias in the context of unit of analysis error, as infants were randomized but some results were provided for individual eyes.

RESULTS

- The rate of recurrence for all subjects was significantly lower with intravitreal bevacizumab (6% versus 26%; odds ratio (OR) 0.17, 95% CI 0.05 to 0.53, $p = 0.002$). The rate of recurrence for subjects with zone I disease was significantly lower with bevacizumab (6% versus 42%; OR 0.09, 95% CI 0.02 to 0.43, $p = 0.03$), but the rate of recurrence with zone II posterior disease did not differ significantly between groups (5% versus 12%; OR 0.39, 95% CI 0.07 to 2.11, $p = 0.27$).
- There were 4 reported cases of ocular complications requiring surgery (1 corneal opacity, 3 lens opacities), all associated with conventional laser therapy. Systemic safety outcomes related to bevacizumab were described in the trial protocol, though were not reported in tables or text.
- Seven infants died before 55 weeks' PMA (5 who underwent intravitreal bevacizumab therapy, 2 who underwent conventional laser therapy). The small numbers preclude the ability to determine whether this difference was due to chance alone.

Criticisms and Limitations: While the BEAT-ROP trial showed a substantial reduction in the recurrence rate of stage 3+ zone I ROP, the authors acknowledge that safety is of tantamount importance for the use of bevacizumab, which the study was not powered to demonstrate. Reporting of safety outcomes that were prespecified in the study protocol was incomplete, and the study lacked long term follow-up for neurodevelopmental outcomes. Since publication of the BEAT-ROP trial results, the dose of bevacizumab used in the trial has also been questioned, in conjunction with concerns regarding safety. A recently published dose-finding study has suggested that a dose 150 times less than the dose used in the BEAT-ROP trial (0.004 mg vs 0.625 mg) may still provide efficacy.[2]

The study was also at significant risk for performance bias. While independent ROP experts were used to review retinal images, the authors describe limitations to blinding those ophthalmologists to prior treatments, due to visible scaring in the eye secondary to laser therapy. However, blinding of neonatal providers could have been achieved (though with some difficulty due to the prevalence of general anesthesia for laser therapy), which could have minimized concerns regarding performance bias.

Other Relevant Studies and Information:
- Pharmacokinetic studies have found anti-VEGF antibodies circulating in the serum of infants treated with bevacizumab, and observational studies have suggested possible concern for adverse pulmonary and neurodevelopmental effects of bevacizumab therapy.[3–5]
- Meta-analysis of randomized trials comparing efficacy of bevacizumab to conventional laser therapy show a consistent reduction in recurrence rate for zone I disease, though no significant reduction in the risk of more serious retinal complications (complete or partial retinal detachment, corneal opacity requiring transplant, cataract removal). There continues to be an absence of long-term safety data regarding delayed systemic effects and neurodevelopmental outcomes among randomized trials.[6]
- Despite the lack of safety data included in the BEAT-ROP trial (and other trials of anti-VEGF therapy), the use of bevacizumab grew substantially after publication. In a retrospective cohort study including data from 48 US children's hospitals from 2010 to 2020, anti-VEGF treatment became the predominant therapy in 2015. Since that time, approximately 70% of patients receiving therapy for ROP annually receive anti-VEGF treatment.[3]
- In addition to lower doses of bevacizumab potentially providing better safety profiles (while maintaining efficacy), alternative VEGF inhibitors with different pharmacokinetics need consideration. Two-year outcomes from a randomized trial of ranibizumab, a monoclonal antibody fragment with a shorter systemic half-life, were recently reported with promising safety outcomes.[7]

Summary and Implications: The BEAT-ROP trial showed a significant reduction in the recurrence rate of stage 3+, zone I ROP, but failed to show a reduction in recurrence of zone II posterior disease and was not powered to assess the safety of bevacizumab. Since publication, observational studies have shown the substantial use of anti-VEGF inhibitors in clinical practice for ROP therapy, with a concurrent increase in the number of adverse effects, including neurodevelopmental outcomes. Awaiting proof from trials are promising advances in the use of anti-VEGF inhibition for ROP therapy, including significant dose reductions from the original trial and alternative inhibitors with more favorable pharmacokinetics.

A CONVERSATION WITH THE TRIALIST: KATHLEEN KENNEDY

Why was long-term follow up performed and reported for only one site?

The bevacizumab study was performed with minimal funding. Most of the participating sites were not academic centers. There was no developmental follow-up prescribed by the study protocol. The one site that reported long-term follow-up was a site that had an existing follow-up program funded by the NICHD Neonatal Research Network.

What might be relative risks: benefits in the under-resourced world given the explosion of ROP there?

If resources are limited such that laser therapy equipment is not available but expertise to administer bevacizumab is, then infants with stage 3+ ROP in Zone I or posterior Zone II could benefit by having ROP therapy available vs not available. The potential risks of bevacizumab, which still have not been fully explored, might be more easily justified in such settings.

Your conclusion was that "this trial was too small to assess safety" yet we see an explosion of use of anti-VEGF agents worldwide. How should your trial have influenced practice or dictated the research agenda?

When this trial was planned and implemented, the use of bevacizumab for ROP was already increasing in the US and elsewhere. That was the impetus for this trial. In an ideal world, a larger trial with long-term follow-up would have been funded and completed before bevacizumab use became widespread. I think it is unfortunate that it is so much more difficult and expensive to properly study new treatments than it is to adopt off-label use of available products.

References

1. Mintz-Hittner HA, Kennedy KA, Chuang AZ; the BEAT-ROP Cooperative Group. Efficacy of intravitreal bevacizumab for stage 3+ retinopathy of prematurity. *N Engl J Med.* 2011;17(364):603–15.
2. Wallace DK, Kraker RT, Freedman SF, et al. Short-term outcomes after very low-dose intravitreous bevacizumab for retinopathy of prematurity. *JAMA Ophthalmol.* 2020;138(6):698–701.
3. Nitkin CR, Bamat NA, Lagatta J, et al. Pulmonary hypertension in preterm infants treated with laser vs anti-vascular endothelial growth factor therapy for retinopathy of prematurity. *JAMA Ophthalmol.* 2022;140(11):1085–1094.
4. Kaushal M, Razak A, Patel W, et al. Neurodevelopmental outcomes following bevacizumab treatment for retinopathy of prematurity: a systematic review and meta-analysis. *J Perinatol.* 2021;41:1225–35.

5. Sato T, Wada K, Arahori H, et al. Serum concentrations of bevacizumab (Avastin) and vascular endothelial growth factor in infants with retinopathy of prematurity. *Am J Ophthalmol.* 2012;153(2):327–33.

6. Sankar MJ, Sankar J, Chandra P. Anti-vascular endothelial growth factor (VEGF) drugs for treatment of retinopathy of prematurity. *Cochrane Database Syst Rev.* 2018;1:CD009734.

7. Marlow N, Stahl A, Lepore D, et al. 2-year outcomes of ranibizumab versus laser therapy for the treatment of very low birthweight infants with retinopathy of prematurity (RAINBOW extension study): prospective follow-up of an open label, randomised controlled trial. *Lancet Child Adolesc Heal.* 2021;5(10):698–707.

Neurology

37

Long-term Effects of Indomethacin Prophylaxis in Extremely Low Birth Weight Infants

The TIPP Trial

WILLIAM MCGUIRE AND PETER W. FOWLIE

"... indomethacin prophylaxis should not be prescribed with the expectation that the chances of survival without neurosensory impairment will be improved."

—SCHMIDT ET AL.[1]

Research Question: Among extremely low birth weight (ELBW) newborn infants, does prophylactic treatment with intravenous indomethacin started within 6 hours of birth versus placebo reduce the risk of death or adverse neurodevelopmental outcomes at 18 months' CA?

Why Was This Study Done: Prior to TIPP, it was known that prophylactic indomethacin reduces the risk of severe intraventricular hemorrhage in ELBW infants, but it was uncertain if this short-term benefit outweighed the risks of drug-induced reductions in cerebral blood flow on long-term neurologic development.

Year Study Began: 1996

Year Study Published: 2001

Study Location: Canada, United States, Hong Kong, New Zealand, and Australia (32 centers total)

Who Was Studied: Infants with birth weights 500 g to 999 g

Who Was Excluded: Infants with structural heart disease, renal disease, congenital abnormalities likely to affect life expectancy or neurodevelopment, thrombocytopenia, overt bleeding at more than one site, hydrops, exposure to maternal indomethacin or another prostaglandin inhibitor within 72 h before birth; infants considered to be "non-viable."

How Many Patients: 1202

Study Overview: The TIPP (Trial of Indomethacin Prophylaxis in Preterms) trial was a parallel-group, masked RCT (Figure 37.1).

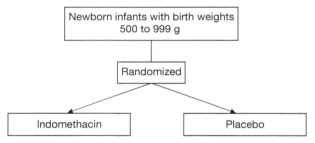

Figure 37.1 Study Overview

What Were the Interventions:
- Infants randomized to the intervention received indomethacin dosed at 0.1 mg/kg every 24 hours for 3 doses starting between 2 and 6 hours after birth.
- Infants randomized to the placebo group received an equal volume of normal saline placebo.

How Long Was Follow-up: 18 months' CA

What Were the Endpoints:
Primary outcome: Composite outcome of death or any of: cerebral palsy (CP), cognitive delay, hearing loss requiring amplification, or bilateral blindness at 18 months' CA.

Selected secondary outcomes: Common complications of prematurity (including PDA, BPD, NEC, IVH, and ROP).

Concerns Regarding Bias: This trial was at overall low risk of bias.

RESULTS

- The primary composite outcome of death, CP, cognitive delay, deafness, or blindness at 18 months' CA occurred in 47% of infants in the indomethacin group versus 46% in the placebo group (odds ratio [OR] 1.1, 95% CI 0.8 to 1.4, $p = 0.61$).
- There was no evidence of between-group differences for any of the individual components of the composite primary outcome.
- Among secondary outcomes, infants in the indomethacin group were less likely to develop a persistent PDA (24% versus 50%; OR 0.3, 95% CI 0.2 to 0.4, $p < 0.001$), or to require subsequent indomethacin therapy or surgical duct ligation. The risk of severe periventricular hemorrhage or IVH, but not of other intracranial abnormalities seen on cerebral ultrasound, was reduced in the indomethacin group (9% versus 13%; OR 0.6, 95% CI 0.4 to 0.9, $p = 0.02$).
- The investigators did not find evidence of effects on other outcomes including BPD, NEC, and bilateral ROP. However, it is notable that the observed point estimate for BPD favored placebo (OR 1.2, 95% CI 0.9 to 1.5, $p = 0.26$), despite a halving of the PDA rate.

Criticisms and Limitations: The TIPP investigators assessed neurodevelopmental outcomes in 95% of the surviving infants at 18 months' CA. Assessors remained unaware of the treatment-group assignments. More than one-quarter of all the surviving infants had moderate-to-severe cognitive delays, defined as a Bayley Scales of Infant Development, Second Edition (BSID-II) Mental Development Index score <70. These scales, however, may not be strongly predictive of school-age behavioral outcomes or later cognitive functioning.[2]

An incremental cost-effectiveness study was performed retrospectively, which did not provide an economic justification for the use of indomethacin prophylaxis for preventing death and neurodevelopmental disabilities in ELBW infants.[3]

Shared decisions about the use of indomethacin prophylaxis for ELBW infants may therefore vary depending on setting, context, and parental and caregiver views, concerns, and expectations. For example, some may value the finding that prophylactic indomethacin reduces the frequency of PDA and severe IVH,[4] particularly where infants need to be transferred to specialist centers for assessment or treatment.

Other Relevant Studies and Information:
- Prior to TIPP, most RCTs of prophylactic indomethacin for very or extremely low birth weight infants assessed short-term (in-hospital) outcomes, such as PDA or IVH.[5] These trials, furthermore, were limited by small sample size and incomplete ascertainment. In addressing this evidence-gap, TIPP provided an unbiased assessment of neurodevelopmental outcomes in a population of ELBW infants who were at high risk of mortality or disability.
- The European consensus guidelines on the management of respiratory distress syndrome do not recommend routine use of prophylactic indomethacin for ELBW infants.[6] It has been suggested that prophylactic indomethacin may be appropriate for infants considered to be at very high risk of IVH (such as infants of birth weight <750 g, or gestation <26 weeks).[7] Post hoc analysis by the TIPP investigators did not show evidence of benefit in subpopulations of ELBW infants with additional risk factors of for severe IVH; however, the absolute risk reduction will be greater in NICUs with high baseline risks of severe IVH.[8]

Summary and Implications: This major collaborative effort showed that it is possible to conduct large, pragmatic trials to resolve important uncertainties in neonatology. The TIPP investigators showed that prophylactic indomethacin is unlikely to increase survival without neurological disability in this population of vulnerable infants.

A CONVERSATION WITH THE TRIALIST: BARBARA SCHMIDT

Why did the meaningful short-term treatment benefit of indomethacin prophylaxis fail to translate into improved neurodevelopment? How does TIPP illustrate which therapies require planning of RCTs with a long-term primary outcome?

Several factors determine whether short-term treatment benefits translate into long-term gains. These factors include (1) the prevalence of the short-term outcome,

(2) the size of the treatment effect, (3) the prognostic accuracy of the short-term outcome, and (4) the long-term safety of the intervention.

Severe IVH is not common, and the treatment effect of prophylactic indomethacin on this outcome is modest. In TIPP, the absolute risk reduction was 4%. Thus, better neurodevelopment due to prevention of severe IVH in the indomethacin group could be expected only in a few infants.

Furthermore, the prognostic accuracy of severe IVH and other signs of brain injury on cranial ultrasound is only fair unless it co-occurs with additional morbidities such as BPD and severe ROP. Each of these 3 morbidities is similarly and independently correlated with poor long-term outcome. Prognostic accuracy strongly increases with the count of these 3 morbidities.[1,2]

Most importantly, **we performed TIPP primarily to study the long-term safety of prophylactic indomethacin.** *We wanted to examine whether the treatment benefits outweigh the potential risks of drug-induced reductions in renal, intestinal, and cerebral blood flow. Indomethacin has multiple targets in the body of a preterm infant. We were interested in the net effect of this powerful drug on long-term development. Long-term follow-up is necessary for trials of common neonatal therapies if their safety profile is uncertain. This is especially true for prophylactic therapies because they are given to many infants who will not benefit from the main effect but can still be harmed by side-effects.*

1. Schmidt B, Asztalos EV, Roberts RS, et al. Impact of bronchopulmonary dysplasia, brain injury, and severe retinopathy on the outcome of extremely low-birth-weight infants at 18 months: results from the trial of indomethacin prophylaxis in preterms. *JAMA.* 2003 Mar 5;289(9):1124–9.
2. Schmidt B, Roberts RS, Davis PG, et al. Prediction of late death or disability at age 5 years using a count of 3 neonatal morbidities in very low birth weight infants. *J Pediatr.* 2015 Nov;167(5):982–6.e2.

References

1. Schmidt B, Davis P, Moddemann D, et al. Long-term effects of indomethacin prophylaxis in extremely low birth weight infants. *N Engl J Med.* 2001;344:1966–72.
2. Luttikhuizen dos Santos ES, de Kieviet JF, Königs M, et al. Predictive value of the Bayley scales of infant development on development of very preterm/very low birth weight children: a meta-analysis. *Early Hum Dev.* 2013;89:487–96.
3. Zupancic JA, Richardson DK, O'Brien BJ, et al.; Trial of Indomethacin Prophylaxis in Preterms Investigators. Retrospective economic evaluation of a controlled trial of indomethacin prophylaxis for patent ductus arteriosus in premature infants. *Early Hum Dev.* 2006;82:97–103.
4. AlFaleh K, Alluwaimi E, AlOsaimi A, et al. A prospective study of maternal preference for indomethacin prophylaxis versus symptomatic treatment of a patent ductus arteriosus in preterm infants. *BMC Pediatr.* 2015;15:47.

5. Fowlie PW, Davis PG, McGuire W. Prophylactic intravenous indomethacin for preventing mortality and morbidity in preterm infants. *Cochrane Database Syst Rev.* 2010;2010(7):CD000174.

6. Sweet DG, Carnielli V, Greisen G, et al. European consensus guidelines on the management of respiratory distress syndrome - 2019 update. *Neonatology.* 2019;115:432–50.

7. Hamrick SE, Sallmon H, Rose AT, et al. Patent ductus arteriosus of the preterm infant. *Pediatrics.* 2020;146:e20201209.

8. Foglia EE, Roberts RS, Stoller JZ, et al.; Trial of Indomethacin Prophylaxis in Preterms Investigators. Effect of prophylactic indomethacin in extremely low birth weight infants based on the predicted risk of severe intraventricular hemorrhage. *Neonatology.* 2018;113:183–6.

38

Effects of Morphine Analgesia in Ventilated Preterm Neonates

The NEOPAIN Trial

SOUVIK MITRA

"Pre-emptive morphine infusions did not reduce the frequency of severe IVH, PVL, or death in ventilated preterm neonates."
—ANAND ET AL.[1]

Research Question: Among ventilated preterm infants born at 23 to 32 weeks' gestation, does preemptive opioid analgesia using intravenous morphine infusion, compared with a placebo control or reduce severe IVH, periventricular leukomalacia (PVL), and/or neonatal death in the first month of life?

Why Was This Study Done: At the time of this trial, routine opioid use for pain control in ventilated very preterm infants was recommended practice.[2] A pilot study by this group (NOPAIN)[3] suggested that preemptive morphine analgesia reduced the incidence of poor neurologic outcomes, and a complicated pathophysiology was invoked to justify the therapy.

Year Study Began: 1998

Year Study Published: 2004

Study Location: United States (12 centers), Sweden (2 centers), France (1 center), United Kingdom (1 center)

Who Was Studied: Infants born at 23 to 32 weeks' gestational age (GA), intubated within 72 hours of birth, and who had been ventilated for <8 hours at enrollment.

Who Was Excluded: Infants with major congenital anomalies, birth asphyxia, intrauterine growth retardation, or maternal opioid addiction; and those participating in other clinical trials.

How Many Patients: 898. Of note, the a priori sample size was 940, with no explanation given for the discrepancy.

Study Overview: The NEOPAIN (Neurologic Outcomes and Pre-emptive Analgesia in Neonates) trial was a parallel-group, masked RCT; with randomization stratified by site and GA (Figure 38.1).

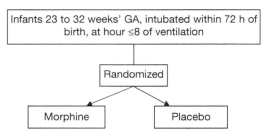

Figure 38.1 Study Overview

What Were the Interventions:
- Infants randomized to the morphine group received a loading dose of morphine (100 µg/kg infused over 1 h); followed by continuous infusions of 10 µg/kg/h for infants born at 23 to 26 weeks' GA, 20 µg/kg/h for infants at 27–29 weeks' GA, or 30 µg/kg/h for infants at 30–32 weeks' GA, up to a maximum of 14 days after initiation of the study drug.
- Infants in the control group received placebo infusions, not further described in the manuscript.

Open-label use of morphine was permitted.

How Long Was Follow-up: 28 to 35 days for infants born ≤30 weeks' GA, or at 14 to 28 days for those born >30 weeks' GA.

What Were the Endpoints:

Primary outcomes: (i) Composite outcome of severe IVH, PVL, and/or neonatal death.

Secondary outcomes: Components of the composite primary outcome, pain response to tracheal suctioning (using Premature Infant Pain Profile (PIPP) scores), days of ventilatory support, days of oxygen supplementation, days to full volume feeding.

Concerns Regarding Bias: The study was at unclear risk of bias in the context of not meeting its goal enrollment. There was attrition bias due to missing cranial ultrasound exams (morphine group 6.7%; placebo group 9.6%).

RESULTS

- There was no difference in the primary composite outcome of severe IVH, PVL, and/or neonatal death between morphine and placebo groups (27% [115/419] versus 26% [105/408]; $p = 0.58$). In addition, there was no difference in its components: severe IVH (13% versus 11%; $p = 0.26$), PVL (7% versus 9%; $p = 0.35$), death (13% versus 11%; $p = 0.25$).
- Fewer infants in the morphine group received open-label treatment compared with the placebo group (45% versus 55%; $p = 0.005$).
- Differences in outcome among infants who received or did not receive open-label morphine were reported, with worse outcomes among those receiving open-label morphine. Additionally, among infants who did not receive open-label morphine, the composite outcome and severe IVH were higher in the morphine group.
- Infants in the morphine group experienced more hypotension after the loading dose ($p = 0.008$) and during the initial 24 hours of drug infusion ($p = 0.0006$). They also required longer duration of mechanical ventilation ($p = 0.03$) and took longer to reach full feeds ($p = 0.0446$).

Criticisms and Limitations: The analysis showed no difference in the composite primary and individual components of the primary outcome. This was one of the first studies that ensured centralized reading of head ultrasounds by an independent radiologist, a feature of strength. However, much has been made of the post hoc exploratory analyses, suggesting harms with open-label morphine use. Although there could be biologic plausibility for such findings, results from post hoc analyses should be interpreted with caution, as the authors emphasize; there could be several reasons for obtaining spurious findings.

First, if a large number of hypotheses are tested post hoc, it is likely that one could obtain a statistically significant result by chance.[4] Second, post hoc hypothesis testing within subsets of the initially randomized population does not guarantee that these subsets remain balanced with respect to known and unknown confounders (i.e., the benefit of randomization and thereby the prognostic balance may be lost).[5] Infants thought to require open-label morphine use were inherently sicker. Therefore, even if a strong association is observed statistically, causality cannot be established.

In this trial, presence of neurological injury such as IVH was not sought prior to initiation of the intervention, though IVH may occur in a vast majority of infants in the first 48 hours of life.[6] Therefore, it is difficult to establish if increased open-label morphine use led to more neurological injury or the resultant irritability from early neurological injury necessitated further opioid use.

Other Relevant Studies and Information:
- The most recent Cochrane update on opioid use for ventilated preterm infants, which was heavily weighted by this trial, shows no difference in neonatal mortality (5 RCTs, $n = 1189$), severe IVH (6 RCTs, $n = 1299$), or PVL (7 RCTs, $n = 1345$); while hypotension requiring medical treatment was significantly higher with opioids (3 RCTs, $n = 1083$).[7]

Summary and Implications: Because there was an increasing concern that NICU procedures were painful, this trial was much anticipated. The NEOPAIN trial demonstrated that preemptive intravenous morphine infusion did not reduce the incidence of death, severe IVH, or PVL in ventilated preterm infants. Possible harms uncovered in post hoc secondary analysis preceded a change in practice away from routine use of opioid infusion for ventilated preterm infants.

A CONVERSATION WITH THE TRIALIST: SUNNY ANAND

Can you give us your thoughts on why the results of your pilot trial, NOPAIN, were not replicated in the larger NEOPAIN trial? What are the resulting implications for trial planning?

Three main reasons may explain the discrepancy in results between the NOPAIN and NEOPAIN trials. First, many improvements occurred in NICU care from

1994–95 (NOPAIN) to 2000–2002 (NEOPAIN) that were primarily directed towards improving the neurologic outcomes of prematurity, which lowered the incidence of early mortality, severe IVH, and severe PVL (or white matter damage) and improved the overall outcomes for all preterm babies, including those in the placebo group. Second, increasing knowledge of and heightened concerns for recurrent neonatal pain, perhaps associated with the detrimental outcomes reported in NOPAIN, caused many NICU providers to give additional, open-label morphine analgesia in NEOPAIN. The increased frequency of morphine doses given as intravenous boluses potentially overdosed some neonates and also caused intermittent hemodynamic instability (opioid vagotonic effect) by lowering the heart rate and blood pressure of preterm neonates. Some neonates may have required IV fluid boluses or vasoactive drugs to overcome these effects, which also increased their risk for developing poor neurologic outcomes, probably more so in the Morphine group. Third, though the morphine dosing regimens for NOPAIN and NEOPAIN were based on single-dose pharmacokinetic studies of morphine, it became very clear that the context-sensitive terminal half-life of morphine was markedly prolonged in preterm neonates receiving continuous infusions.[1] Consequently, we found extremely high morphine levels in the NEOPAIN trial coupled with delayed morphine clearance in preterm neonates,[2] which was accentuated in newborns with decreased gut motility.[1–3]

For planning a new randomized trial, I recommend using significantly lower loading doses and infusion rates of morphine (or fentanyl), regulate the therapy based on objective measures of neonatal pain (not observer-dependent), mandate strict and specific criteria for administering additional analgesia (e.g., high pain score, instead of the "clinician preferences" used in NEOPAIN) and use an adaptive trial design. Also, instead of ventilated preterm neonates, future trials should include post-surgical neonates experiencing continuous postoperative pain for 24–48 hours.[4]

1. Saarenmaa E, Neuvonen PJ, Rosenberg P, et al. Morphine clearance and effects in newborn infants in relation to gestational age. *Clin Pharmacol Ther.* 2000;68:160–6.

2. Anand KJS et al. Morphine pharmacokinetics and pharmacodynamics in preterm and term neonates: secondary results from the Neopain Trial. *Br J Anaesth.* 2008;101:680–9.

3. Menon G et al. Morphine analgesia and gastrointestinal morbidity in preterm infants: secondary results from the Neopain Trial. *Arch Dis Child Fetal Neonatal Ed.* 2008;93:F362–7.

4. Kinoshita M, Stempel KS, Borges do Nascimento IJ, et al. Systemic opioids versus other analgesics and sedatives for postoperative pain in neonates. *Cochrane Database Syst Rev.* 2023;3:CD014876.

References

1. Anand KJS, Hall RW, Desai N, et al. Effects of morphine analgesia in ventilated pre-term neonates: primary outcomes from the NEOPAIN randomised trial. *Lancet.* 2004 May 22;363(9422):1673–82.
2. Anand KJ; International Evidence-Based Group for Neonatal Pain. Consensus state-ment for the prevention and management of pain in the newborn. *Adolesc Med.* 2001;155(2):173–80.
3. Anand KJ, Barton BA, McIntosh N, et al. Analgesia and sedation in preterm neonates who require ventilatory support: results from the NOPAIN trial. Neonatal Outcome and Prolonged Analgesia in Neonates. *Arch Pediatr Adolesc Med.* 1999 Apr;153(4):331–8.
4. Li G, Taljaard M, Van den Heuvel ER, Levine MA, et al. An introduction to multi-plicity issues in clinical trials: the what, why, when and how. *Int J Epidemiol.* 2017 Apr 1;46(2):746–55.
5. Lee YJ, Ellenberg JH, Hirtz DG, et al. Analysis of clinical trials by treatment actually received: is it really an option? *Stat Med.* 1991 Oct;10(10):1595–605.
6. Ballabh P. Intraventricular hemorrhage in premature infants: mechanism of disease. *Pediatr Res.* 2010 Jan;67(1):1–8.
7. Bellù R, Romantsik O, Nava C, et al. Opioids for newborn infants receiving mechan-ical ventilation. *Cochrane Database Syst Rev.* 2021 Mar 17;3:CD013732.

39

Whole-Body Hypothermia for Neonates with Hypoxic-Ischemic Encephalopathy

WES ONLAND AND ANTON H. VAN KAAM

"Our findings demonstrate the safety and effectiveness of whole-body cooling in reducing the risk of death or disability among infants with moderate or severe encephalopathy."
—SHANKARAN ET AL.[1]

Research Question: Does whole-body cooling initiated before 6 hours of life and continued for 72 hours in infants ≥36 weeks' gestation with moderate to severe HIE reduce death or disability at 18 to 22 months of age as compared with infants given standard care?

Why Was This Study Done: Prior to this trial, there was no effective treatment for reducing the high risk of death or severe neurodevelopmental impairment for infants with hypoxic ischemic encephalopathy (HIE).

Year Study Began: 2000

Year Study Published: 2005

Study Location: United States (15 centers)

Who Was Studied: Infants ≥36 weeks' gestation <6 hours of age who met criteria establishing risk for perinatal asphyxia (metabolic acidosis pH ≤7.0 in the first hour of life; or acute perinatal event; and a 10-minute Apgar score of 5 or less *or* assisted ventilation at birth continuing for at least 10 minutes) and evidence of moderate or severe HIE on a standardized neurologic exam.

Who Was Excluded: Infants with chromosomal or major congenital abnormalities, severe growth restriction (birthweight ≤1800 g), or for whom no further aggressive treatment was planned.

How Many Patients: 208

Study Overview: This trial was a parallel-group, masked RCT (Figure 39.1).

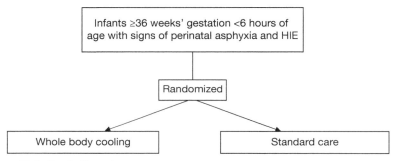

Figure 39.1 Study Overview

What Were the Interventions:
- Infants randomized to servo-controlled whole-body cooling were placed on an infant-size blanket (Blanketrol II Hyper-Hypothermia System, Cincinnati Sub-Zero). The esophageal target temperature, as measured by an inserted probe, was 33.5°C. After 72 hours of hypothermia, the set point of the automatic control on the cooling system was slowly increased by 0.5°C per hour to a goal of 36.5°C.
- Infants randomized to standard care had target skin temperatures maintained by servomechanism between 36.5 and 37.0°C initially, followed by usual care at each center.

How Long Was Follow-up: 18 to 20 months

What Were the Endpoints:

Primary outcome: Composite outcome of death or moderate or severe disability at 18 to 22 months. Moderate or severe disability was defined as any of the following found by certified neurologic assessment: a Mental Development Index score of the Bayley Scales of Infant Development-Second Edition (BSID-II) more than one standard deviation below the mean score, a Gross Motor Function Classification System grade of level 2 to 5, hearing impairment with or without requiring hearing aids, blindness, or a persistent seizure disorder. Different degrees of cognitive impairment, gross motor impairment, and hearing and vision loss were used to distinguish between moderate and severe disability.

Selected secondary outcomes: Cardiac arrhythmia, persistent acidosis, major-vessel thrombosis or bleeding, skin changes, hypotension, length of stay.

Concerns for Bias: The trial was at high risk for performance/detection bias, as caregivers were not blinded to the intervention. However, certified neurologic assessments for both eligibility and for primary outcome reduced this issue, as did the blinding of follow-up examiners to the treatment assignment.

RESULTS

- Infants receiving therapeutic hypothermia had a reduced risk of death or moderate or severe disability at 18 to 22 months (44% versus 62%; relative risk [RR] 0.72; 95% CI 0.54 to 0.95; $p = 0.01$).
- No significant difference was found in any individual component of the composite primary outcome. Twenty-four percent of the infants died in the hypothermia group, and 37% in the control group (RR 0.68, 95% CI 0.44 to 1.05, $p = 0.08$).
- The incidence of serious adverse events was similar in the hypothermia and standard care groups.

Criticisms and Limitations: Lack of blinding might introduce a potential bias, especially as death is a component of the primary outcome, and withdrawal of intensive care treatment was the leading cause of death in this study. Of the infants who died, 50% had support withdrawn in the hypothermia group, compared with 71% in the standard care group. A recent systematic review summarizing

119 RCTs in critical care medicine showed that treatment effects for blinded studies are smaller than for unblinded studies: therefore, the unblinded intervention design of this study should be taken into account when interpreting the results.[2]

Another debatable issue of this trial is the assessment of suspected HIE and degree of encephalopathy. Although the study listed clear inclusion criteria for study entry and included a training and certification process for neurologic assessments, some of the chosen criteria might not be objective enough. Blood gas analysis can give false positive and negative results, and assessment of Apgar scores and level of encephalopathy have a low interrater reliability.[3] Future research should investigate if more objective parameters, such as amplitude integrated electroencephalogram or biomarkers, can more reliably identify patients at risk of poor neurodevelopmental outcome following perinatal asphyxia.[4]

Other Relevant Studies and Information:
- Meta-analysis combining this trial and 10 other RCTs showed that therapeutic hypothermia significantly reduced the risk of the composite outcome of death or major neurodevelopmental disability to 18 months (typical RR 0.75, 95% CI 0.68 to 0.83; number needed to treat 7) and its separate components without severe adverse effects.[5]
- The results of this trial led the International Liaison Committee on Resuscitation (ILCOR) to recommend adoption of this treatment for all NICUs.[6]
- The generalizability to low- and middle-income countries was recently questioned by a large RCT in India, Sri Lanka, and Bangladesh; which demonstrated no reduction in the combined outcome of death or disability at 18 months with therapeutic hypothermia, but an increase in death (See HELIX, Chapter 44).[7]

Summary and Implications: This trial showed that therapeutic hypothermia is effective in reducing in the composite outcome death or moderate or severe neurodevelopmental disability in term or near-term infants with HIE. The results of this trial led to widespread introduction of therapeutic hypothermia as standard of care in this high-risk population. Many NICUs used the design of this trial as guidance for their hypothermia protocol.

A CONVERSATION WITH THE TRIALIST: SEETHA SHANKARAN

How do you hope to help provide the evidence base that will support/refute the "therapeutic creep" evident in current practice? What are your thoughts on future trials of milder HIE and later cooling?

Regarding offering cooling mild HIE, neither safety nor efficacy has been demonstrated yet, but there is one RCT and a comparative effectiveness trial, both ongoing in this country that will provide information in the future. An RCT of hypothermia versus targeted normothermia has just been funded in the UK; I am involved in that trial. Of course, it will be 5 years before the results are available.

Regarding initiating cooling after 6 hours of age, the NICHD Neonatal Research RCT did demonstrate possibility of benefit (Bayesian analysis), for infants with moderate or severe HIE when initiated between 6 and 24 hours of age. I think talking to families and offering cooling for these infants is a good approach.

A sizeable percentage of the infants in the control group had temperatures above normal range. Have you estimated the treatment difference between the 2 groups that may be attributed to excess temperature in the control group rather than cooling in the intervention group?

This is an excellent question and we at NICHD NRN did not do this, so I cannot give you an answer. Many of us have talked about a future [individual] patient data analysis that may assess this question. I can say that the trials in the high-income countries (all enrolling participants in late 1990s, early 2000s), had 14%–38% of infants with at least one episode of elevated temperature in the control group. This was before it was recognized that elevated temperature increased risk of adverse outcome. The trials all showed direction of benefit of cooling, however.

References

1. Shankaran S, Laptook AR, Ehrenkranz RA, et al. Whole-body hypothermia for neonates with hypoxic-ischemic encephalopathy. *New Engl J Med.* 2005;353(15):1574–84.
2. Baiardo Redaelli M, Belletti A, Monti G, et al. The impact of non-blinding in critical care medicine trials. *J Crit Care.* 2018;48:414–7.
3. Tagin MA, Gunn AJ. Neonatal encephalopathy and potential lost opportunities: when the story fits, please cool. *Arch Dis Child Fetal Neonatal Ed.* 2021;106(5):458–9.
4. Shankaran S, Laptook A, Thayyil S. Hypothermia for neonatal encephalopathy: how do we move forward? *Arch Dis Child Fetal Neonatal Ed.* 2022;107(1):4–5.

5. Jacobs SE, Berg M, Hunt R, et al. Cooling for newborns with hypoxic ischaemic en-cephalopathy. *Cochrane Database Syst Rev*. 2013(1):CD003311.

6. Hoehn T, Hansmann G, Buhrer C, et al. Therapeutic hypothermia in neonates. review of current clinical data, ILCOR recommendations and suggestions for implementa-tion in neonatal intensive care units. *Resuscitation*. 2008;78(1):7–12.

7. Thayyil S, Pant S, Montaldo P, et al. Hypothermia for moderate or severe neo-natal encephalopathy in low-income and middle-income countries (HELIX): a randomised controlled trial in India, Sri Lanka, and Bangladesh. *Lancet Glob Health*. 2021;9:e1273–85.

40

Effectiveness of Sucrose Analgesia in Newborns Undergoing Painful Medical Procedures

DAVID OSBORN

"Based on these results, we recommend using sucrose to reduce pain in newborns undergoing venipuncture for the newborn screening test but not for intramuscular injection of vitamin K. In addition, sucrose is not recommended for heel lances for glucose monitoring in newborns of diabetic mothers."

—TADDIO ET AL.[1]

Research Question: In healthy term or late preterm newborn infants of diabetic and nondiabetic mothers, does oral sucrose, as compared with placebo, reduce pain during intramuscular injection of vitamin K, venipuncture for the newborn screening test, and heel lance for blood glucose monitoring without serious adverse effects?

Why Was This Study Done: At the time of this study, pain management guidelines promoted the widespread use of sucrose. However, only few painful procedures had been evaluated, and concerns remained that sucrose may raise blood glucose levels in newborns of diabetic mothers.

Year Study Began: 2003

Year Study Published: 2008

Study Location: Canada (single center)

Who Was Studied: Healthy newborns (≥36 weeks' gestation) born to nondiabetic mothers with uneventful pregnancies or to diabetic mothers (type 1, type 2, or gestational diabetes controlled by diet or insulin).

Who Was Excluded: Newborns with major congenital or neurologic anomalies, or clinical diagnoses of birth asphyxia or seizures; newborns admitted to the NICU, those who received analgesics and/or sedatives, or those scheduled to undergo circumcision during the study period.

How Many Patients: 240

Study Overview: This study was a parallel-group, masked RCT; stratified by diabetic or nondiabetic mother (Figure 40.1).

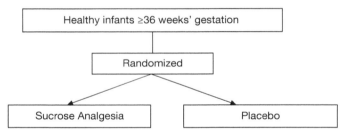

Figure 40.1 Study Overview

What Were the Interventions:
- Infants randomized to sucrose analgesia received 2 mL of a 24% sucrose solution by mouth before all intramuscular injections, venipunctures, and heel-lances performed within 2 days of birth.
- Infants randomized to placebo received an equal volume of sterile water by mouth.

How Long Was Follow-up: Pain scores were measured during procedures. Monitoring for adverse events lasted 30 minutes post-procedure.

What Were the Endpoints:
Primary outcome: Pain, measured using the validated Premature Infant Pain Score (PIPP) from video recording of procedure.

Selected secondary outcomes: Physiologic responses including heart rate and oxygen saturation. Recorded adverse events included "spitting up" and blood glucose levels in infants or diabetic mothers.

Concerns Regarding Bias: This study was at overall low risk of bias.

RESULTS

- In the analysis of all infants undergoing a painful procedure, the pain was lower among newborns who received sucrose (mean difference [MD] – 1.3; 95% CI –2.0 to –0.6, p <0.001).
- During venipuncture, newborns who received sucrose had lower pain scores (newborns of nondiabetic mothers: MD –3.2; 95% CI –4.6 to –1.8, p <0.001; newborns of diabetic mothers: MD –2.4; 95% CI –3.8 to –1.0, p <0.001).
- In infants receiving an intramuscular injection, pain did not differ significantly between the sucrose and placebo groups for newborns of diabetic or nondiabetic mothers (newborns of nondiabetic mothers: MD –1.1; 95% CI –2.4 to 0.2, p = 0.10; newborns of diabetic mothers: MD –1.0; 95% CI –2.4 to 0.4, p = 0.15).
- Pain scores among newborns of diabetic mothers undergoing heel lance did not differ between the sucrose and placebo groups (MD 0; 95% CI - 1.2 to 1.1, p = 0.94).
- Among newborns of diabetic mothers, there was no difference in the incidence of minor adverse effects or mean blood glucose levels. Among newborns of nondiabetic mothers, more newborns in the placebo group spat up. There were no serious adverse events during the study.

Criticisms and Limitations: This trial provides reliable evidence for the short-term efficacy and safety of sucrose for common minor procedural pain in healthy newborn infants of nondiabetic and diabetic mothers. However, the study does not report longer-term effects of repeated sucrose exposure in newborn infants.

Despite the study reporting numbers in excess of the sample size calculation, the PIPP score estimates of effect have greater imprecision than predicted. Certainty of evidence for non-efficacy should be downgraded, particularly for intramuscular injections.

Other Relevant Studies and Information:
- Although there are at least 74 studies enrolling 7049 infants, the Cochrane systematic review[2] of sucrose for analgesia in newborn infants

is limited due to the variability of indications, sucrose concentrations, and co-interventions studied, with the largest comparison including only 343 infants. The review found that sucrose is effective for reducing procedural pain from single events such as heel lance, venipuncture, and intramuscular injection in both preterm and term infants. No serious side effects or harms were documented with this intervention. Taddio et al. was the only included trial that reported no difference in blood glucose levels in infants of diabetic mothers undergoing repeated heel lance monitoring.

- The American Academy of Pediatrics update on prevention and management of procedural pain in the neonate policy statement recommended that oral sucrose and/or glucose solutions can be effective in neonates undergoing mild to moderately painful procedures, either alone or in combination with other pain relief strategies.[3]
- Further studies of sucrose analgesia are warranted, including sucrose use in combination with other interventions, use in extremely preterm and/or unstable infants, dose optimization, and the effect of repeated administration on short- and long-term outcomes.
- Other substrates such as breastfeeding or breast milk feeding could present an alternative means of pain control.[4]

Summary and Implications: This trial provides reliable evidence for the short-term efficacy and safety of sucrose for common minor procedural pain in healthy newborn infants of nondiabetic and diabetic mothers. The use of sucrose should be incorporated into strategies for reducing pain and stress in infants of nondiabetic and diabetic mothers undergoing mild to moderately painful procedures.

A CONVERSATION WITH THE TRIALIST: ANNA TADDIO

What do you hope to see in future studies on pain management for the neonate?

More non-invasive care, involvement of parents/caregivers, more evaluation of interventions.

The ethics of pain control studies in the neonate were carefully considered by your study team, with use of a placebo control determined to be necessary given unanswered questions on effectiveness. Can you give us any insight into the discussions around this decision, as sucrose analgesia was already widely used at the time of this study?

Our consideration was clinical equipoise. The therapy was not in use. In our community, there was consensus that there was insufficient data that addressed all important aspects of evaluation of this therapy. Ethical considerations are important discussions to have when planning any study, in particular, those involving placebos.

With now >70 studies addressing the use of sucrose for neonates undergoing painful procedures, the only reports we have are on physiologic outcomes and pain scores. What are your thoughts on the studies to address longer-term behavioral or growth issues?

Unfortunately, there are few studies that address "long-term" outcomes, and they are hard to do. At this point, observational designs may be the most feasible and acceptable approaches to address these outcomes.

References

1. Taddio A, Shah V, Hancock R, et al. Effectiveness of sucrose analgesia in newborns undergoing painful medical procedures. *CMAJ: Canadian Medical Association Journal = journal de l'Association medicale canadienne.* 2008;179:37–43.
2. Stevens B, Yamada J, Ohlsson A, et al. Sucrose for analgesia in newborn infants undergoing painful procedures. *Cochrane Database Syst Rev.* 2016;7(7):CD001069.
3. Committee on Fetus and Newborn and Section on Anesthesiology and Pain Medicine. Prevention and management of procedural pain in the neonate: an update. *Pediatrics.* 2016;137:e20154271.
4. Shah PS, Herbozo C, Aliwalas LL, et al. Breastfeeding or breast milk for procedural pain in neonates. *Cochrane Database Syst Rev.* 2012;12(12):CD004950.

41

A Randomized Trial of Prenatal Versus Postnatal Repair of Myelomeningocele

The MOMS Trial

SARA B. DEMAURO

"Prenatal surgery for myelomeningocele reduced the need for shunting and improved motor outcomes at 30 months, but the early intervention was associated with both maternal and fetal morbidity."
—ADZICK ET AL.[1]

Research Question: Among infants with a prenatal diagnosis of myelomeningocele, does prenatal repair, as compared to postnatal repair, lead to reduced mortality or need for cerebrospinal fluid (CSF) shunt in the first year, and improved neurodevelopment at 30 months?

Why Was This Study Done: Prior to this trial, at least 200 mother–baby dyads had already undergone prenatal surgery for repair of myelomeningocele without clear evidence that the benefits of this procedure outweighed the risks.

Year Study Began: 2003

Year Study Published: 2011

Study Location: United States (3 maternal–fetal surgery centers)

Who Was Studied: Singleton pregnancies in which the fetus had a myelomeningocele with the upper boundary of the defect between T1 and S1 vertebral bodies, evidence of hindbrain herniation, a gestational age of 19 0/7 to 25 6/7 weeks, and a normal karyotype.

Who Was Excluded: Infants with fetal anomalies unrelated to the myelomeningocele, severe kyphosis, risk of preterm birth, placental abruption, maternal body mass index ≥35, or other maternal contraindication to surgery.

How Many Patients: MOMS was terminated early for increased efficacy in the intervention group after a planned interim analysis at both the 12- and 30-month timepoints. When the trial was stopped, 183 out of a planned 200 patients had been recruited.

Study Overview: MOMS was a parallel-group, masked, RCT (Figure 41.1).

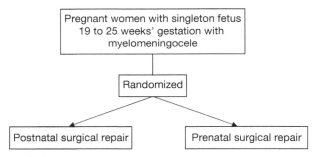

Figure 41.1 Study Overview

What Were the Interventions:
- Infants randomized to the prenatal surgery group underwent prenatal myelomeningocele repair.
- Infants in the postnatal repair group underwent myelomeningocele repair after birth by the same group of surgeons.

How Long Was Follow-up: 12 and 30 months

What Were the Endpoints:
Primary outcomes: Composite outcome of fetal or neonatal death or the need for a CSF shunt at 12 months. Composite outcome of Bayley II Mental Development Index (MDI) and adjusted motor function level at 30 months.
Selected secondary outcomes: Pregnancy and surgical complications, child developmental outcomes.

Concerns Regarding Bias: Surgical trials entail a high risk for bias in ascertainment of outcomes because it is difficult to blind the intervention. To mitigate this risk, the MOMS investigators used rigorous approaches to blind personnel responsible for determining all study outcomes. Additional bias may be present with early termination of study enrollment.

RESULTS

- Although 183 women were randomized, the MOMS publication includes 12-month outcomes for the 158 mother–infant dyads who were randomized before July 1, 2009 and 30-month outcomes for the 134 dyads who were randomized before December 1, 2007.
- Fetal or neonatal death or need for a CSF shunt by the age of 12 months occurred in 68% of the prenatal surgery group and 98% of the postnatal surgery group (relative risk 0.7, 97.7% confidence interval [CI] 0.58 to 0.84, p <0.01). Shunt placement was less common with prenatal surgery (40% versus 82%; RR 0.48, 95% CI 0.36 to 0.64, p <0.001), but the incidence of death before shunt placement was slightly higher (3% versus 0%).
- In the prenatal surgery group, birthing women had higher rates of oligohydramnios, premature rupture of the membranes, membrane separation, and receipt of blood transfusion; and one-third had thinning or dehiscence of the hysterotomy scar at delivery. Further, 13% delivered before 30 weeks, as compared to 0% in the postnatal group.
- At 30 months, children in the prenatal surgery group had better developmental outcomes, which was attributable to a significant improvement in adjusted motor function level, or the difference between a child's functional level and anatomic level of lesion. There was no difference in MDI scores between the 2 groups.
- Notable secondary outcomes in the children included lower rates of hindbrain herniation (64% versus 96%; relative risk 0.67, 95% CI 0.56 to 0.81, p <0.001) and higher likelihood of independent walking at 30 months (42% versus 21%; relative risk 2.01, 95% CI 1.16 to 3.48, p = 0.01) in the prenatal surgery group.

Criticisms and Limitations: A key limitation is that the successes reported in MOMS were achieved by a small number of highly subspecialized, multidisciplinary teams. Subsequent literature demonstrated that at least 35 cases for standard hysterotomy to more than 56 cases for newer minimally invasive approaches must be performed for surgeons to achieve competency in this procedure.[2] Therefore, it remains best performed by limited numbers of teams with sufficient training and experience.

A second consideration is that the trial was stopped early, before enrollment of the full target sample size. While the interim evidence of efficacy placed an ethical mandate to stop early, it is also known that such truncated trials can produce more extreme results. This potential bias may have been amplified by the, also justifiable, early and incomplete reporting prior to the outcomes of the full enrolled cohort.

Finally, investigators applied a rigorous set of eligibility criteria when screening for the trial; ultimately, 16.8% of screened women were randomized. This approach to identification of eligible study participants limits the generalizability of MOMS. Whether the benefits and risks are equivalent when this procedure is utilized in mothers and infants with different baseline characteristics is uncertain. To address these questions, the North American Fetal Therapy Network has developed a Fetal Myelomeningocele Consortium and outcomes registry (NAFTNet.org).

Other Relevant Studies and Information:
- Given the uncertainty at the time, Adzick and colleagues were able to convince surgeons at all other maternal–fetal surgery centers in the United States to *not* offer experimental prenatal repair while the trial was underway. This is an unusual example of *equipoise* in the medical community.
- As noted above, the MOMS trial did not report the outcomes for all dyads randomized. A full report of the 12-month outcomes was consistent with the primary paper.[3] In a full report of 30-month outcomes, prenatal surgery improved the composite outcome of mental development and motor function as well as several secondary outcomes including independent ambulation, but did not improve cognitive development.[4]

Summary and Implications: MOMS moved fetal surgery from being a procedure only considered for life-threatening conditions to a procedure that may be considered to mitigate the adverse effects of lesions not uniformly life-limiting. This approach to myelomeningocele repair decreased the risk of death or need for CSF shunt at 12 months and improved motor function at 30 months. On balance, women treated with prenatal surgery had higher rates of pregnancy complications and were more likely to deliver preterm.

A CONVERSATION WITH THE TRIALIST: SCOTT ADZICK

Prenatal surgery for myelomeningocele is not a cure. I repeat, it is not a cure.
—Scott Adzick, Hot Topics Conference 2019

How did your team approach the trade-off of incomplete data on the long-term outcomes with the certain knowledge that prenatal repair created more very preterm and extremely preterm infants?

Prior to the start of the MOMS trial in 2003, we had preliminary data on more than 200 cases of fetal surgery for myelomeningocele from the 3 participating centers: UCSF, Vanderbilt, and CHOP. There seemed to be some benefits from the prenatal surgery, but clearly preterm delivery was one of the complications. We shared this information with potential MOMS trial participants, and we had equipoise when counseling them.

References

1. Adzick NS, Thom EA, Spong CY, et al. A randomized trial of prenatal versus postnatal repair of myelomeningocele. *N Engl J Med*. 2011;364(11):993–1004.
2. Joyeux L, De Bie F, Danzer E, et al. Learning curves of open and endoscopic fetal spina bifida closure: systematic review and meta-analysis. *Ultrasound Obstet Gynecol*. 2020;55(6):730–39.
3. Tulipan N, Wellons III JC, Thom EA, et al. Prenatal surgery or myelomeningocele and the need for cerebrospinal fluid shunt placement. *J Neurosurg Pediatr*. 2015;16:613e20.
4. Farmer DL, Thom EA, Brock JW 3rd, et al.; Management of Myelomeningocele Study Investigators. The Management of Myelomeningocele Study; full cohort 30-month pediatric outcomes. *Am J Obstet Gynecol*. 2018;218(2):256.

42

Neurodevelopmental Outcome at 5 Years of Age After General Anesthesia or Awake-Regional Anesthesia in Infancy

The GAS Trial

SARA B. DEMAURO

"The GAS trial . . . provides strong evidence that just under one hour of general anesthesia in infancy does not cause significant neurocognitive or behavioral deficits."

—McCann et al.[1]

Research Question: Do children exposed to awake-regional anesthesia versus general anesthesia during inguinal hernia surgery as infants have equivalent neurodevelopmental outcomes at 5 years?

Why Was This Study Done: Prior large cohort studies had suggested associations between general anesthesia in infancy or early childhood and behavioral problems or poor academic achievement. Evidence for an effect on IQ was less consistent.[2] This was the first RCT to assess the effect of general anesthesia in infancy on childhood neurocognitive outcomes.

Year Study Began: 2007

Year Study Published: 2019

Study Location: Australia, Italy, United States, United Kingdom, Canada, Netherlands, and New Zealand (28 centers total)

Who Was Studied: Infants born after 26 weeks' gestation and before 60 weeks' PMA at the time of enrollment, undergoing inguinal herniorrhaphies.

Who Was Excluded: Prior exposure to general anesthesia or contraindication to awake-regional or general anesthesia, congenital heart disease, mechanical ventilation before surgery, known chromosomal abnormalities or other congenital abnormalities that could affect neurodevelopment, known neurologic injury, anticipated difficulty with follow-up, or neurodevelopmental assessment not available in child's anticipated primary language.

How Many Patients: 722 infants were randomized; 719 were retained for the intention to treat analysis.

Study Overview: The GAS (General Anaesthesia or Awake-Regional Anaesthesia in Infancy) trial was a parallel-group, randomized controlled, equivalence trial (Figure 42.1).

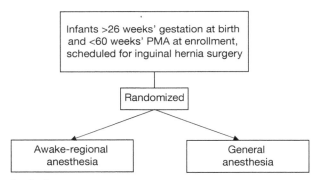

Figure 42.1 Study Overview

What Were the Interventions:
- Infants randomized to awake-regional anesthesia received a spinal, caudal, or combined caudal/spinal anesthetic according to institutional preferences.
- Infants randomized to general anesthesia received sevoflurane-based general anesthesia.

How Long Was Follow-up: 5 years

What Were the Endpoints:
Primary outcome: Wechsler Preschool and Primary Scale of Intelligence-3rd Edition (WPPSI-III) full scale intelligence quotient (FSIQ) at 5 years of age.
Secondary outcomes: Additional outcomes measured at 5 years were executive functions, school readiness skills, adaptive function, behavior, and neurodevelopmental or neurosensory impairments.

Concerns Regarding Bias: The study was at unclear risk of performance/detection bias, as surgeons and anesthesiologists were not blinded to the intervention and about half of parents were aware of their child's treatment. In addition, the randomized assignment was discovered by the study pediatrician in about 4.0% of cases and by the psychologist in about 2.5% of cases.
The study was also at unclear risk of attrition bias. Per protocol, the primary analysis excluded children for whom regional anesthesia failed. In addition, attrition was higher than anticipated; thus, the primary complete case data, as-per-protocol analysis included only 62% of the enrolled children.

RESULTS

- Regional anesthesia was unsuccessful in 19%, all of whom were converted to general anesthesia.
- The WPPSI-III FWIQ scores at 5 years were equivalent in children exposed to general and awake-regional anesthesia, with an adjusted mean difference of 0.23 (95% CI –2.59 to 3.06) points in the as-per-protocol analysis. This result met the investigators' a priori definition of equivalence because the 95% confidence interval fell completely within ± 5 points.
- Secondary outcomes were equivalent in as-per-protocol and intention-to-treat analyses, with and without multiple imputation.

Criticisms and Limitations: Complete case data for the primary outcome at 5 years were only available for 62% of children randomized in the GAS trial. The authors performed multiple imputation to resolve missing data including missing outcomes. Unfortunately, missing developmental outcomes cannot easily be predicted. It is unknown whether children lost to follow-up have higher or lower risk for developmental problems.[3,4] McCann et al. report that children lost to follow-up at 5 years were more likely to have performed poorly on the 2-year assessment. However, significant differences between 2-year developmental assessments and 5-year cognitive assessments in high-risk preterm populations are well documented.[5,6] This limitation is a reminder to incorporate rigorous strategies to limit attrition in trials that require longitudinal follow-up.

Despite its attrition, the GAS trial provides insight into the likely safety of short-term anesthesia during infancy to assist clinical decision-making. However, it does not answer questions about longer exposures, exposure to multiple agents, or multiple episodes of anesthesia. Therefore, this trial should not be generalized to those potentially higher-risk clinical scenarios. In addition, most participants were preterm males, possibly limiting generalizability to other groups of infants.

A final limitation of the GAS trial is related to the sample size. Some prior large cohort studies had suggested associations between general anesthesia and neurobehavioral problems such as ADHD.[2] GAS was not powered or reported with sufficiently long follow-up to detect differences in such problems, so the possibility of these effects cannot be completely ruled out with the existing trial data. Nevertheless, GAS still provides the least biased estimates of such impacts that are available to date.

Other Relevant Studies and Information:
- Interim analysis of the GAS trial was published 3 years before the primary trial manuscript. The investigators reported equivalent performance on the Bayley Scales of Infant and Toddler Development, 3rd Edition, at 2 years of age between children exposed to regional versus general anesthesia in infancy.[7]
- The Cochrane Library published a review of regional versus general anesthesia for preterm infant herniorrhaphy in 2015.[8] Fewer than 140 infants were included, and only short-term/perioperative outcomes were reported. The authors called for a large RCT such as GAS.

Summary and Implications: GAS was the first RCT to compare regional versus general anesthesia during infancy, addressing concerns for long-term developmental harm from general anesthesia based on observational studies. The investigators demonstrated equivalence of the 2 approaches—both IQ and all secondary neurodevelopmental outcomes were similar in the 2 study arms. Based on these results, clinicians and parents can be reassured that a single short exposure to general anesthesia during infancy likely does not have adverse developmental consequences during childhood.

A CONVERSATION WITH THE TRIALIST:
ANDREW J. DAVIDSON, SENIOR AUTHOR

Do you think an RCT of longer-term surgery-anesthesia is possible? What considerations would you make for the control arm for such a study?

There definitely need to be more trials to determine the optimal anesthetic and peri-operative management strategies in neonates and infants. Many neonates having major surgery have a poor outcome. This may be due to many factors that are not necessarily related to anesthesia neurotoxicity. The control arm would depend on what aspect of management we are comparing and within that what strategies we are comparing – blood pressure management, cerebral oxygenation, ventilation strategies, fluid management, etc. The questions in the trials would be based on what we can glean from more detailed observational studies and from the biology and basic principles behind the questions. As such quite a bit of work needs to be done before we can do these trials.

As far as neurotoxicity studies, one comparator arm would be an increasingly opioid-based technique similar to the TREX trial [NCT03089905] which is underway and compares remifentanil/dexmedetomidine/low dose sevoflurane to standard dose sevoflurane. These trials can't get underway until we understand more about the pharmacology of anaesthesia in infants and especially neonates. There is work underway to determine a more robust measure of anesthesia effect in this age group. Once this is done, we can move further into comparing different regimens.

References

1. McCann ME, de Graaff JC, Dorris L, et al.; GAS Consortium. Neurodevelopmental outcome at 5 years of age after general anaesthesia or awake-regional anaesthesia in infancy (GAS): an international, multicentre, randomized, controlled equivalence trial. *Lancet.* 2019;393(10172):664–77.
2. Davidson AJ, Sun LS. Clinical evidence for any effect of anesthesia on the developing brain. *Anesthesiology.* 2018;128:840–53.
3. Guillén U, DeMauro S, Ma L, et al. Relationship between attrition and neurodevelopmental impairment rates in extremely preterm infants at 18 to 24 months: a systematic review. *Arch Pediatr Adolesc Med.* 2012;166(2):178–84.
4. Aylward GP, Hatcher RP, Stripp B, et al. Who goes and who stays: subject loss in a multicenter, longitudinal follow-up study. *J Dev Behav Pediatr.* 1985;6:3–8.
5. Marlow N, Wolke D, Bracewell MA, et al.; EPICure Study Group. Neurologic and developmental disability at six years of age after extremely preterm birth. *N Engl J Med.* 2005;352(1):9–19.

6. Schmidt B, Anderson PJ, Doyle LW, et al.; Caffeine for Apnea of Prematurity (CAP) Trial Investigators. Survival without disability to age 5 years after neonatal caffeine therapy for apnea of prematurity. *JAMA*. 2012 Jan 18;307(3):275–82.
7. Davidson AJ, Disma N, de Graaff JC, et al.; GAS consortium. Neurodevelopmental outcome at 2 years of age after general anaesthesia and awake-regional anaesthesia in infancy (GAS): an international multicentre, randomised controlled trial. *Lancet*. 2016;387:239–50.
8. Jones LJ, Craven PD, Lakkundi A, et al. Regional (spinal, epidural, caudal) versus general anaesthesia in preterm infants undergoing inguinal herniorrhaphy in early infancy. *Cochrane Database Syst Rev*. 2015;(6):CD003669.

43

Levetiracetam Versus Phenobarbital for Neonatal Seizures

The NEOLEV2 Trial

STEFAN JOHANSSON

"In this study conducted . . . with near real-time response to continuous video EEG monitoring, phenobarbital was more effective than
levetiracetam in achieving seizure cessation."

—SHARPE ET AL.[1]

Research Question: Among late preterm and term infants with neonatal
seizures of any etiology, is levetiracetam compared with phenobarbital superior
as the first-line treatment, in achieving absence of continuous electroencephalog-
raphy (cEEG) documented seizures for at least 24 hours?

Why Was This Study Done: At the time of this trial, levetiracetam had already
been incorporated into clinical practice for management of neonatal seizures,
ahead of prospective evidence of its efficacy in neonates.[2] Moreover, therapy with
phenobarbital had been questioned for side effects and for failure to stop seizures.

Year Study Began: 2013

Year Study Published: 2020

Study Location: United States (5 centers), New Zealand (1 center)

Who Was Studied: Infants at 36 to 44 weeks' PMA, <2 weeks postnatal age, and weighing ≥2.2 kg. It was intended that only those with EEG-confirmed seizures would be recruited.

Who Was Excluded: Infants given any previous anticonvulsants (excepting short-acting benzodiazepines), with serum creatinine levels >1.6 mg/dL (>141 micromol/L), with seizures related to correctable metabolic or electrolyte disturbances, or for whom death was imminent.

How Many Patients: 106 infants were randomized, of whom 83 infants were included in modified intention-to-treat analyses. The target sample size was 100 infants, with an allocation ratio of 60:40 levetiracetam versus phenobarbital.

Study Overview: NEOLEV2 trial (Efficacy of Intravenous Levetiracetam in Neonatal Seizures) was a parallel-group, masked, phase IIb, RCT (Figure 43.1).

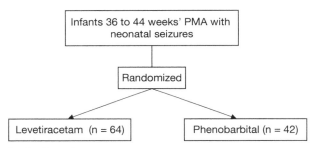

Figure 43.1 Study Overview

What Were the Interventions:
- Infants randomized to levetiracetam received an initial dose of 40 mg/kg levetiracetam, followed by an additional 20 mg/kg dose if seizures persisted.
- Infants randomized to phenobarbital received an initial dose of 20 mg/kg, followed by an additional 20 mg/kg dose if seizures persisted.

Both drugs were administered per a dose-escalation regimen, and with crossover to the other drug in case of treatment failure.

How Long Was Follow-up: Up to 48 hours

What Were the Endpoints:
Primary outcome: Electrographic seizure freedom for 24 hours.
Selected secondary outcomes: Electrographic seizure freedom for 48 hours, seizure freedom for one hour, subgroup-analyses of the primary outcome measure for subjects with HIE.

Concerns Regarding Bias: The study was at serious risk of attrition bias, given the exclusion of 23 infants with missing data in the modified intention-to-treat analyses. Additional bias may have been introduced with the redefinition of the primary outcome (from 48 hour seizure free period to 24 hour period) after recruitment was completed. The level of company personnel involvement may also have introduced bias.

RESULTS

- A larger proportion of infants treated with phenobarbital became seizure free for 24 hours (80% versus 28%; RR 0.35, 95% CI 0.22 to 0.56, p <0.001).
- Subgroup analysis of patients treated with hypothermia for HIE demonstrated similar efficacy results.
- A 7.5% improvement in efficacy was achieved with a dose escalation of levetiracetam from 40 to 60 mg/kg.
- Rates of any adverse effects (including hypotension, respiratory suppression, and sedation) were more common in the phenobarbital group, although not statistically significant (31% versus 19%; relative risk 0.61, 95% CI 0.31 to 1.20).

Criticisms and Limitations: Efficacy studies of anticonvulsants for neonatal seizures need to be carefully designed, especially when it comes to diagnosing occurrence of seizures and defining seizure control. The NEOLEV2 trial protocol was well designed in this respect. All infants were monitored with continuous video EEG. For inclusion in the intention-to-treat analyses, neurophysiologists were to confirm seizures before treatment and validate seizure control after treatment. While this was stated as a strict requirement for inclusion, it was not applied until after randomization, which meant that 23 of 106 randomized infants were not included in the "modified" intention-to-treat analyses.

Another limitation was the change of the primary outcome after patient recruitment was completed, from 48 to 24 hours of seizure freedom. The reason was that many infants had their EEG monitoring discontinued before 48 hours due to clinically indicated investigations or transfer to another hospital. According to the investigators, this change did not introduce bias. However, an alternative approach would have been to keep 48 hours of seizure freedom as the primary outcome as originally planned, and present 24 hours of seizure freedom as a secondary endpoint. Reassuringly, both the 24-hour and 48-hour epochs had similar efficacy rates in favor of phenobarbital.

The findings of the NEOLEV2 trial are not easy to generalize to many real-world NICUs, where infants with clinical seizures are often treated with anticonvulsants before electrographic confirmation by a neurophysiologist, if such a service is even available. Compared to this RCT, a regular clinical context includes infants given anticonvulsant drugs due to "seizures" without EEG signs, while other infants with electrographic seizures are not treated in the absence of clinical signs. To assess the safety of drugs like phenobarbital and levetiracetam, a more pragmatic trial design with a large study population would be needed. Efficacy and safety endpoints beyond 48 hours of life should be a key feature of such a trial.

Other Relevant Studies and Information:
- The findings in the NEOLEV2 trial align with a recent network meta-analysis, suggesting phenobarbital be used as first-line treatment.[3]
- Another recent meta-analysis suggests that levetiracetam is associated with fewer side-effects compared to phenobarbital.[4]

Summary and Implications: The NEOLEV2 trial showed that phenobarbital was more effective than levetiracetam in achieving 24 hours of seizure freedom in late preterm and term infants, possibly at the expense of more side-effects such as hypotension and sedation. Given the careful definition of seizures and short-term seizure control in this trial, it is hard to generalize findings regarding efficacy and safety to many NICUs. Furthermore, the NEOLEV2 trial does not guide treatment decisions for outcomes beyond 48 hours. A large and more pragmatically designed study with long-term endpoints is warranted.

A CONVERSATION WITH THE TRIALIST:
RICHARD HAAS

How relevant are cEEG outcomes, as compared to long-term clinically more robust outcomes?

We do not yet have robust evidence that aggressive cEEG monitoring and treatment aimed at elimination of seizure activity with ASM's improves long-term neurodevelopmental outcome. The definitive study to address this must wait until we have antiseizure medications with good safety and efficacy in seizure cessation that are not themselves neurotoxic. If such a study were undertaken currently using current standard of care treatments for neonatal seizures, (phenobarbital, phenytoin, and benzodiazepines) any neurodevelopmental benefit of seizure cessation might be negated by the neurotoxic effects of the medications themselves.

Can you explain your choice to modify the intention to treat analysis?

Intention to treat analyses are emphasized as preferable in clinical trial design. In NEOLEV2 our chosen primary endpoint was seizure cessation verified by 2 independent neurophysiologist[s], that is, a modified intention to treat analysis.

The new diagnostic framework for neonatal seizures emphasizes the key role of EEG in diagnosis of neonatal seizures,[1] that is, seizures are defined electrographically.

Neonatal cEEG data is difficult to interpret, and experts frequently differ in how they interpret it. We wanted the most accurate and robust measure of seizures and seizure cessation possible.

In the mITT analysis, data was excluded for patients who had been treated because the neurologist at the bedside reading the EEG in real-time diagnosed seizures, but on review the independent neurophysiologists did not agree that definite seizure activity was present pre-treatment. In addition, some cEEG records were unavailable for neurophysiologist review. These data would have been included in a pragmatic trial using an intention to treat analysis.

1. Pressler RM, Cilio MR, Mizrahi EM, et al. The ILAE classification of seizures and the epilepsies: Modification for seizures in the neonate. Position paper by the ILAE Task Force on Neonatal Seizures. *Epilepsia*. 2021;62(3):615-28.

References

1. Sharpe C, Reiner GE, Davis SL, et al. Levetiracetam versus phenobarbital for neonatal seizures: a randomized controlled trial. *Pediatrics*. 2020;145(6):e20193182.
2. Silverstein FS, Ferriero DM. Off-label use of antiepileptic drugs for the treatment of neonatal seizures. *Pediatr Neurol*. 2008;39(2):77–9.
3. Xu ZE, Li WB, Qiao MY, et al. Comparative efficacy of anti-epileptic drugs for neonatal seizures: A network meta-analysis. *Pediatr Neonatol*. 2021;62(6):598–605.
4. Hooper RG, Ramaswamy VV, Wahid RM, et al. Levetiracetam as the first-line treatment for neonatal seizures: a systematic review and meta-analysis. *Dev Med Child Neurol*. 2021;63:1283–93.

44

Hypothermia for Moderate or Severe Neonatal Encephalopathy in Low-Income and Middle-Income Countries

The HELIX Trial

SRINIVAS MURKI

"These findings do not support the routine use of therapeutic hypothermia for all infants with moderate to severe asphyxia from low income and middle income countries."

THAYYIL ET AL.[1]

Research Question: For full-term babies with moderate or severe neonatal encephalopathy who have been admitted to tertiary neonatal units in low- and middle-income countries (LMICs), does therapeutic hypothermia reduce death or disability at 18 to 22 months when compared with standard care?

Why Was This Study Done: Therapeutic hypothermia reduces death or disability after neonatal encephalopathy in high-income countries. However, prior to this trial, evidence on the efficacy or safety of therapeutic hypothermia in LMICs was lacking.

Year Study Began: 2015

Year Study Published: 2021

Study Location: India (5 centers), Sri Lanka (1 center), Bangladesh (1 center)

Who Was Studied: Infants ≥36 weeks' gestation with birthweight ≥1800 g in the first 6 hours of life who had both 1) evidence of perinatal depression at 5 min of life; either by requiring resuscitation, receiving an Apgar ≤6, or, for home births, demonstrating an absence of crying by 5 minutes and 2) evidence of moderate to severe encephalopathy.

Who Was Excluded: Infants who had no heart rate at 10 minutes of life despite adequate resuscitation, those with major life-threatening congenital malformations, or whose parents were unable to attend follow-up.

How Many Patients: 408

Study Overview: The HELIX (hypothermia for neonatal encephalopathy in LMICs) trial was a parallel-group, unmasked RCT (Figure 44.1).

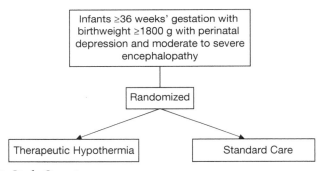

Figure 44.1 Study Overview

What Were the Interventions: Babies allocated to the hypothermia group had a controlled reduction of their rectal temperature to 33.5°C for 72 h, followed by automated re-warming at 0.5°C per h with the use of a servo-controlled whole-body cooling device. Control group infants had usual neonatal intensive care.

How Long Was Follow-up: 18 to 22 months

What Were the Endpoints:
Primary outcome: Composite outcome of death or moderate to severe disability. Severe disability was defined as any one of the following: cognitive composite score ≤70 based on the Bayley Scales of Infant and Toddler Development, Third

Edition (BSID-III) (conducted in home languages), gross motor function classification system level 3–5, hearing impairment requiring hearing aids or cochlear implant, or blindness. Moderate disability was defined as cognitive composite score (BSID-III) of 70 to 84 and one or more of the following: gross motor function classification system level 2, hearing impairment with no amplification, or persistent seizure disorder.

Selected secondary outcomes: Death or major morbidities prior to hospital discharge, or at 18 to 22 months; MRI (magnetic resonance imaging) biomarkers.

Concerns Regarding Bias: There was high risk for performance/detection bias, as caregivers were not blinded to the intervention. However, those who assessed neurodevelopment and MRIs were blinded.

RESULTS

- The risks of death or moderate to severe disability were similar in the therapeutic hypothermia and standard care groups (50% versus 47%; RR 1.06, 95% CI 0.87 to 1.30, $p = 0.55$).
- Therapeutic hypothermia increased the risk of death by 18 months (42% versus 31%; RR 1.35, 95% CI 1.04 to 1.76, $p = 0.022$).
- Infants in the hypothermia group had more coagulopathy, gastric bleeds, cardiac arrythmia, severe thrombocytopenia, persistent metabolic acidosis, persistent hypotension, and a longer hospital stay.
- MRI evidence of brain injury and sepsis did not differ between the groups.

Criticisms and Limitations: The increase in death in treated infants came as a surprise given the results of previous trials, and led to strong statements regarding withholding therapeutic hypothermia from current care in NICUs in the LMIC setting. While concern is understandable, the interpretation and generalizability of these results demands more inspection.

The trial demonstrated appropriate therapeutic hypothermia technique; however, the question of to whom this therapy was applied is troubling. It is likely in this trial that the population in question was a sicker and more chronically ill group. Entry criteria did not require any reporting of antepartum sentinel events, and many of the infants studied were born at home with limited ability to monitor or assess. Additionally, MR imaging of the study cohort suggest a subacute or partial prolonged hypoxic insult, contrary to the images reported in other trials that reported perinatal insults. This suggests the etiology of HIE in this population was quite different from that of the population studied in well-resourced countries, and requires differing strategies. Perhaps a trial of therapeutic hypothermia of infants in the LMIC setting who only met the strictest of criteria for perinatal depression would have demonstrated different results. Abandonment of this potentially life-saving technique is not the answer, but hurdles remain in the LMIC setting for identifying the population who will benefit.

Other Relevant Studies and Information:
- A recent meta-analysis, including a total of 28 RCTs (representing 3592 infants), suggested a reduction in mortality with therapeutic hypothermia to infants with moderate to severe encephalopathy, as well as a greater benefit to infants in low-income countries on subgroup analysis.[2]
- Considering the existing evidence and the results of the HELIX trial, a position statement from National Neonatology Forum (NNF) India provides guidance on the use of therapeutic hypothermia.[3] It recommends therapeutic hypothermia for neonates with gestational age ≥36 weeks and <6 hours of life, with perinatal depression and evidence of moderate to severe encephalopathy; with therapeutic hypothermia to be administered only at qualifying level III or IV facilities.

Summary and Implications: The HELIX trial highlights the need for more research on therapeutic hypothermia in LMICs, and the importance of adopting therapeutic hypothermia as a therapy only for infants with HIE with strictly defined population characteristics and only in units with adequate staff expertise and follow-up facilities.

A CONVERSATION WITH THE TRIALIST: SUDHIN THAYYIL

Approaching consent for this trial was likely quite an undertaking. Could you discuss the consent issues that you dealt with?

Very little is known about the complexities of informed parental consent for neonatal trials in LMIC. In a systematic review of parental consent rates for neonatal intervention trials, we found that parental consent rates in LMIC, particularly in India, were much higher than in high-income countries (96% versus 83%). Ironically, we were concerned about high rather than low consent rates—we were worried that parents from low socioeconomic back grounds may not understand research nor would be empowered to decline trial participation.

In the HELIX trial, we used a series of measures for effective and informed parental consenting. Firstly, specific training was given to the clinical team and research nurses to avoid any coercion or inducement, and to ensure participation was fully voluntary. We then video recorded the consenting process and analysed these videos for quality assurance under 3 domains – empathy, information, and autonomy. Finally, we also conduced qualitative interviews of the clinicians and parents to review their views and experiences of the consenting process. These issues have been published separately,[1] but the key observations were: 1) clinicians did provide all key information prior to consenting, although they tried to not use the term "clinical trial" due to the stigma associated with this term in India; 2) parents consented primarily based on the trust they had in the physicians and possible therapeutic misconception; 3) involvement of extended family was vital and choice was often made by paternal family members; 4) parents very much appreciated the efforts of the research nurses, who acted as a bridge between the health care facilities.

How can we best identify who might best benefit from cooling?

This is a very difficult issue. Clinical trials are rarely powered for subgroup analysis. Using magnetic resonance biomarkers, we could not identify any subgroup in the HELIX trial who benefitted from cooling. It was harmful at all the participating sites, and ineffective both amongst inborn and outborn babies, although the harm was much higher amongst outborn babies. Exploring why cooling did not work in LMIC is likely to be more useful in developing future neuroprotective therapies, than identifying a small subgroup who might benefit.

1. Pant S, Elias MA, Woolfall K, et al. Parental and professional perceptions of informed consent and participation in a time-critical neonatal trial: a mixed-methods study in India, Sri Lanka and Bangladesh. *BMJ Glob Health* 2021;6(5):e005757.

References

1. Thayyil S, Pant S, Montaldo P, et al. Hypothermia for moderate or severe neonatal encephalopathy in low-income and middle-income countries (HELIX): a randomised controlled trial in India, Sri Lanka, and Bangladesh. *Lancet Glob Health*. 2021;9(9):e1273–85.
2. Abate BB, Bimerew M, Gebremichael B, et al. Effects of therapeutic hypothermia on death among asphyxiated neonates with hypoxic-ischemic encephalopathy: A systematic review and meta-analysis of randomized control trials. *PLoS One*. 2021 Feb 25;16(2):e0247229.
3. Position Statement and Guidelines for Use of Therapeutic Hypothermia to Treat Neonatal Hypoxic Ischemic Encephalopathy In India, National Neonatology Forum of India (personal communication).

Intrapartum Care

45

A Controlled Trial of Antepartum Glucocorticoid Treatment for Prevention of the Respiratory Distress Syndrome in Premature Infants

SARAH D. MCDONALD

"... there is sufficient evidence of beneficial effects on lung function and of absence of adverse effects to justify further trials [with betamethasone]. In view of the present trial's empirical basis of selection of glucocorticoid and its dosage and duration of treatment, it would be surprising if there were no scope for improved results from therapeutic regimens based on a better understanding of the mode of action of glucocorticoids...."
—LIGGINS ET AL.[1]

Research Question: In pregnant people admitted in preterm labor at 24 to 36 weeks' gestation, or in whom preterm delivery is planned before 37 weeks because of an obstetrical complication, do 2 doses administered 24 hours apart of: 1) 12 mg betamethasone compared with 2) an identical-appearing control of 6 mg cortisone acetate (<2% the potency), reduce the incidence of neonatal respiratory distress syndrome (RDS) in the first week of life?

Why Was This Study Done: This study followed an animal study of parturition by Liggins, in which he observed that lambs exposed to antenatal corticosteroids in an experimental model of preterm labor had increased survival and improved lung expansion.[2]

Year Study Began: 1969

Year Study Published: 1972

Study Location: New Zealand (single center)

Who Was Studied: Infants of pregnant people admitted in preterm labor at 24 to 36 weeks' gestation or in whom delivery was planned before 37 weeks because of an obstetrical complication (including congenital fetal malformation, Rh isoimmunization, maternal preeclampsia ["hypertension-edema-proteinuria syndromes"], and placental previa). Singletons, twins, and triplets were mentioned.

Who Was Excluded: Mother–infant dyads for whom an obstetrician considered corticosteroid treatment to be contraindicated or delivery occurred soon after admission.

How Many Patients: Of 287 randomized patients, 282 pregnant people with at least 295 fetuses were included; 172 infants were delivered ≥24 hours after trial entry.

Study Overview: This trial was a parallel-group, masked RCT (Figure 45.1).

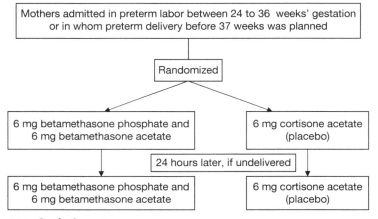

Figure 45.1 Study Overview

What Were the Interventions:
- Pregnant people randomized to the betamethasone group received an intramuscular injection of a mixture of 6 mg betamethasone phosphate and 6 mg betamethasone acetate.
- Pregnant people randomized to the placebo group received an intramuscular injection of an identical-appearing control of 6 mg cortisone acetate.

Unless delivery had already occurred, a second injection was administered 24 hours later of the same substance initially given.

How Long Was Follow-up: Duration was not explicitly stated in the article.

What Were the Endpoints:

Primary outcome: Respiratory distress syndrome (RDS); defined as clinical signs of grunting, chest retractions present during the first 3 hours and persisting beyond the first 6 hours after birth, <u>and</u> a radiological pattern having fine generalized granularity of the lung fields with air bronchograms.
Selected secondary outcomes: Perinatal mortality (fetal death or death within the first 7 days), intraventricular hemorrhage.

Concerns Regarding Bias: This early trial was published in the era prior to CONSORT reporting standards. The reporting of all outcomes was on subsets of data rather than all infants (including the primary outcome which was reported in less than 90% of infants), and the extent to which other interventions were used in the 2 groups was not reported (e.g., tocolysis with ethanol or salbutamol, antibiotics, amniocentesis).

RESULTS

- There were 5 categories of pregnant patients included, the majority being the preterm labor group ($n = 213$, 76%; with 226 infants), in whom approximately 23% in each group delivered <24 hours after entry into the trial, and presumably did not receive the second dose.
- The primary outcome of RDS was reported in a total of 263 liveborn infants (out of at least 295 infants), born after preeclampsia, preterm labor, and Rh isoimmunization: 12/143 (8.4%) in the betamethasone group and 31/120 (25.8%) in the control group. Outcomes were not reported in

the other 2 categories (placenta previa and major fetal anomalies, which were the indication for entry in a total of 16 women, with an unreported number of infants).

- The outcome of perinatal death (fetal death or death within the first 7 days) was reported for 279 infants (after preeclampsia, unplanned preterm labor, and Rh isoimmunization): 16/153 (10.4%) in the betamethasone group and 25/126 (19.8%) in the control group. After unplanned preterm labor, intraventricular hemorrhage was not present in any of the infants in the betamethasone group and 5.3% in the control group (not significant); this data was derived from postmortem examination, so it applies to a subset of infants, given that the trial was conducted before routine neonatal head ultrasound.

Criticisms and Limitations: This landmark trial was conducted between 1969 and 1972, before the CONSORT reporting standards were published. As such, information that is now standard was not included, such as a table reporting baseline characteristics of mothers or infants. Maternal enrollment criteria were broad, but ultimately 76% of mothers enrolled due to threatened preterm delivery. The report mostly focuses on this subpopulation. A sample size calculation was not included, but the very large difference in RDS points to more than adequate power if outcomes in the 2 other subgroups of infants were similar as that presented in the 3 subgroups.

Other Relevant Studies and Information:
- The updated 2020 Cochrane review[3] includes this trial and the 26 subsequent RCTs using similar doses of betamethasone or dexamethasone. Findings confirm significant reductions in perinatal death (RR 0.85, 95% CI 0.77 to 0.93; 2.3% fewer), neonatal death (RR 0.78, 95% CI 0.70 to 0.87; 2.6% fewer), and RDS (RR 0.71, 95% CI 0.65 to 0.78; 4.3% fewer), as well as intraventricular hemorrhage and necrotizing enterocolitis.
- There is limited evidence on long-term outcomes and alternate dosing regimens.[4-7]
- Animal evidence suggests the current doses may be 2 to 10 times higher than required.[8]
- A recent systematic review has highlighted that there may be increased risks of long-term harm, including adverse neurocognitive and

psychological outcomes,[9] particularly in the children who are ultimately born at or near term, who, given the challenges of predicting preterm birth, constitute approximately half of those exposed to steroids.[10]

Summary and Implications: Liggins and Howie published the first RCT evaluating antenatal corticosteroids in 1972. The many subsequent trials that followed confirmed their findings that antenatal corticosteroids reduce mortality and morbidity in those preterm infants exposed to steroids.[11] However, it was not until several decades after Liggins and Howie's trial that this powerful therapy was incorporated widely into practice and reflected in clinical practice guidelines.[12,13] Despite the initial urging of Liggins and Howie for dose-finding studies, it has only been recently, after almost 50 years of using ~24 mg of betamethasone or dexamethasone antenatal corticosteroid therapy, that new RCTs[7] undertook examining lower doses of these powerful medications.

A CONVERSATION WITH THE EXPERT: OLIVIER BAUD

Given that approximately half of babies exposed to antenatal corticosteroids in utero exceed expectations and are born at or near term, and mounting evidence of long-term adverse neurocognitive effects in these infants, what should be the clinical approach with steroids?

It's a great question! Actually, we are very inaccurate in selecting a targeted population of women at risk of preterm delivery and therefore eligible for antenatal steroids. I think that we would first need to use the few predictive models to refine who should be treated because delivery is really expected to occur within a few days.

The Liggins study led to many other trials, involving more than 7700 infants, highlighted in Jack Sinclair's cumulative meta-analysis. What opportunities for research questions did we miss in planning and performing those trials (including head-to-head comparisons; alternative (lower) doses; effects in very early and late gestation, and longer-term risk for exposed infants at lower risk?

You're right in suggesting we have missed something in the field. Most of the trials you mentioned are either replicates of Liggins' study or fed the debate about the multiple courses. We have indeed missed major unanswered questions regarding the effect of this treatment on babies born near/full term or regarding dosage adjustment. And finally, considering that a treatment can be given worldwide at the same dosage whatever the number of fetuses, distribution volume of the woman, risk of imminent birth, etc... is quite surprising. The recent trial by Cynthia Gyamfi-Bannerman is a remarkable contribution but it can lead to increase again the risk of exposing fetuses to steroids with relatively limited benefits and (perhaps) long-term adverse effects. The BETADOSE trial, even inconclusive, will certainly have the positive impact of stimulating a new field of research towards precision/individualized medicine in women at risk of preterm infants. I speculate that research in this field is not at all completed!

References

1. Liggins GC, Howie RN. A controlled trial of antepartum glucocorticoid treatment for prevention of the respiratory distress syndrome in premature infants. *Pediatrics.* 1972;50(4):515–25.
2. Liggins GC. Premature delivery of foetal lambs infused with glucocorticoids. *J Endocrinol.* 1969;45(4):515–23.
3. McGoldrick E, Stewart F, Parker R, et al. Antenatal corticosteroids for accelerating fetal lung maturation for women at risk of preterm birth. *Cochrane Database Syst Rev.* 2020;12(12):CD004454.
4. Ninan K, Morfaw F, Murphy KE, et al. Neonatal and maternal outcomes of lower versus standard doses of antenatal corticosteroids for women at risk of preterm delivery: a systematic review of randomized controlled trials. *J Obstet Gynaecol Can.* 2021;43(1):74–81.
5. Senat M, Minoui S, Multon O, et al. Effect of dexamethasone and betamethasone on fetal heart rate variability in preterm labour: a randomised study. *BJOG.* 1998;105(7):749–55.
6. Schmitz T, Alberti C, Ursino M, et al. Full versus half dose of antenatal betamethasone to prevent severe neonatal respiratory distress syndrome associated with preterm birth: study protocol for a randomised, multicenter, double blind, placebo-controlled, non-inferiority trial (BETADOSE). *BMC Pregnancy and Childbirth.* 2019;19(1):67.
7. Schmitz T, Doret-Dion M, Baud O, et al.; BETADOSE Trial Study Group; Groupe de Recherche en Obstétrique et Gynécologie. Neonatal outcomes for women at risk of preterm delivery given half dose versus full dose of antenatal betamethasone: a randomised, multicentre, double-blind, placebo-controlled, non-inferiority trial. *Lancet.* 2022;400(10352):592–604.
8. Jobe AH, Kemp M, Schmidt A, et al. Antenatal corticosteroids: a reappraisal of the drug formulation and dose. *Pediatr Res.* 2021;89:318–25.
9. Ninan K, Liyanage SK, Murphy KE, et al. Evaluation of long-term outcomes associated with preterm exposure to antenatal corticosteroids: a systematic review and meta-analysis." *JAMA Pediatr.* 2022;176(6):e220483.
10. Räikkönen K, Gissler M, Kajantie E. Associations between maternal antenatal corticosteroid treatment and mental and behavioral disorders in children. *JAMA.* 2020;323(19):1924–33.
11. Sinclair JC. Meta-analysis of randomized controlled trials of antenatal corticosteroid for the prevention of respiratory distress syndrome: discussion. *Am J Obstet Gynecol.* 1995;173(1):335–44.

12. National Institute of Child Health and Human Development. Effect of corticosteroids for fetal maturation on perinatal outcomes. NIH Consensus Statement. 1994;12:1–24.

13. Wright LL, Horbar JD, Gunkel H, et al. Evidence from multicenter networks on the current use of antenatal corticosteroids in very low birth weight infants. *American Journal of Obstetrics and Gynecology.* 1995;173(1):263–269.

Prevention of Early-Onset Neonatal Group B Streptococcal Disease with Selective Intrapartum Chemoprophylaxis

MEGAN J. TURNER AND CLYDE J. WRIGHT

"Selective intrapartum chemoprophylaxis is likely to prevent at least 50 percent of the cases of early-onset group B streptococcal disease, and 75 percent of the deaths from the disorder."
—BOYER AND GOTOFF[1]

Research Question: Among mothers with group B *Streptococcus* (GBS) colonization and pregnancy complicated by preterm labor and/or prolonged rupture of membranes, does intrapartum prophylaxis with ampicillin, as compared with no treatment, reduce early-onset neonatal GBS disease?

Why Was This Study Done: At the time of this trial, GBS was responsible for most newborn deaths from early-onset sepsis. In the decade preceding this publication, the authors laid the foundation for this study by describing strategies for eradication of GBS colonization, prophylaxis of GBS disease, and a rationale for selective screening to identify the highest-risk mothers.[2–4]

Year Study Began: 1979

Year Study Published: 1986

Study Location: United States (single center)

Who Was Studied: Mothers with GBS colonization and either preterm labor (<37 weeks) and/or prolonged (>12 hours) rupture of membranes (ROM), and their infants.

Who Was Excluded: Mothers with penicillin allergy or who were treated with other antimicrobials. Mothers in both groups who developed fever after randomization were treated with ampicillin and removed from the study.

How Many Patients: 180 mothers and their 185 infants, but 20 women and their 21 infants were excluded from the analysis.

Study Overview: This was a parallel-group, unmasked RCT (Figure 46.1). In the manuscript, the authors also describe a larger, non-randomized observational cohort study.

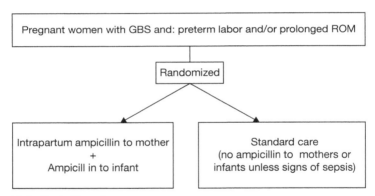

Figure 46.1 Study Overview

What Were the Interventions:
- Women randomized to the intervention group received ampicillin 2 g intravenously (IV) followed by 1 g IV every 4 hours until delivery. Their infants received ampicillin 50 mg/kg every 12 hours until initial culture results were available.
- Women randomized to the control group received no intrapartum antibiotics; if intrapartum fever developed, the women were treated with ampicillin and removed from the study. Control infants did not receive antibiotics unless symptoms were suggestive of sepsis.

How Long Was Follow-up: Hospital discharge

What Were the Endpoints:
Primary outcome: Infant colonization with GBS
Selected secondary outcomes:

- *(Infant)* Colonization at multiple (≥3) sites, GBS bacteremia.
- *(Maternal)* Postpartum GBS colonization, postpartum fever, postpartum GBS disease, side effects necessitating ampicillin discontinuation.

Concerns Regarding Bias: There was potential for bias to be introduced at several points in the study. There was risk for performance/detection bias, as blinding to the study intervention was not performed. The study was also at risk for selective attrition bias, as 13 women were excluded after developing intrapartum fever. Concerns for reporting and other bias have additionally been noted, as this ongoing study was reported on 3 occasions, with communication making it clear that the research team was aware of the study results and continued recruitment until statistical significance had been reached.[5] This was possible since no prior sample size was calculated.

RESULTS

- Intrapartum ampicillin was associated with a 5.6-fold reduction in infant GBS colonization (9% versus 51%; p <0.001), and a 7.5-fold reduction in GBS colonization at ≥3 sites (4% versus 30%; p <0.001).
- Bacteremia occurred in no infants in the treatment group, compared with 6% in the control group (p = 0.024).
- In the 47% of mothers who were evaluated for this secondary outcome, maternal postpartum colonization was decreased nearly four-fold in the treatment group (86% versus 26%; p <0.001). Maternal treatment was associated with only one case of urticaria; no other treatment-limiting events were described.
- In a bold extrapolation of their findings, the authors suggest that "selective intrapartum chemoprophylaxis is likely to prevent at least 50% of the cases of early-onset GBS disease and 75% of the deaths from this disorder." Additionally, in an economic extrapolation, the authors estimate annual savings in the US of $256 million.

Criticisms and Limitations: The authors only report data on in-hospital outcomes on mothers and infants. There is incomplete data on the impact of chemoprophylaxis on maternal colonization, with fewer than half of mothers with postpartum cultures obtained. This substantial rate of missing samples limits the authors' ability to conclude definitively that vaginal colonization was reduced by intrapartum ampicillin. Additionally, they report that there were no cases of late-onset sepsis ($\geq$7 days of life); it is unclear how they would have followed infants for this likely post-discharge complication.

Other Relevant Studies and Information:
- With the publication of Boyer and Gotoff's study, antibiotic chemoprophylaxis became the standard for women with GBS colonization. This led to a sharp decrease in the overall incidence of early-onset sepsis, from 3 to 4 cases per 1000 live births to approximately 0.5 per 1000.[6,7]
- In the 2014 Cochrane review of intrapartum antibiotic prophylaxis (IAP),[8] Ohlsson and Shah analyzed 3 relatively small RCTs evaluating IAP for the prevention of neonatal early-onset GBS infection (including this study; 488 mother-infant pairs total) and reported an overall risk ratio of 0.17 (95% CI 0.04 to 0.74) favoring IAP compared with placebo. However, there were methodologic concerns regarding the included studies.
- In the years following this study, these recommendations have evolved. Current obstetrical recommendations include antibiotic prophylaxis for women with GBS colonization unless a prelabor Cesarean birth is performed in the setting of intact membranes.[9] With the development and implementation of the neonatal early-onset sepsis calculator risk stratification tool,[10] the number of infants receiving antibiotic prophylaxis has substantially decreased, with no evidence of inferiority to conservative management.[11]

Summary and Implications: This study provided evidence for selective intrapartum chemoprophylaxis for early-onset neonatal GBS disease. The investigators sought to expose only the group most likely to experience severe morbidity or mortality from GBS to a prophylactic therapy. In doing so, they demonstrated the utility of a strategy that minimizes cost, side effects, and the risk of drug resistance. Despite serious limitations and multiple risks of bias, this study led the way for IAP practice guidelines and the subsequent dramatic reduction in infant morbidity and mortality from early-onset GBS disease.

A FEW WORDS FROM THE EDITOR

Boyer [and] Gotoff's trial was pivotal in providing the evidence support for an intervention that was quickly and successfully adopted, with a dramatic improvement in the incidence of early-onset sepsis.[1] However, the story of GBS prophylaxis is also a lesson in the need for continual re-evaluation of "proven" treatments, as we cannot fully measure downstream effects of exposure nor anticipate all consequences of practice changes. Given evolving concerns for potential adverse health consequences of altering an infant's microbial balance with antibiotics, the effect of this prophylaxis on the newborn gut microbiota must be a continued area of study. Additionally, consideration of alternatives, including vaccines, is ongoing.[2]

—Susanne Hay and Roger Soll

1. Schrag SJ, Farley MM, Petit S, et al. Epidemiology of invasive early-onset neonatal sepsis, 2005 to 2014. *Pediatrics*. 2016;138(6):e20162013.
2. The American College of Obstetricians and Gynecologists. Committee Opinion: Prevention of Group B streptococcal early-onset disease in newborns. *ACOG Clinical*. 2023;https://www.acog.org/clinical/clinical-guidance/committee-opinion/articles/2020/02/prevention-of-group-b-streptococcal-early-onset-disease-in-newborns

References

1. Boyer KM, Gotoff SP. Prevention of early-onset neonatal group B streptococcal disease with selective intrapartum chemoprophylaxis. *NEJM*. 1986;314(26):1665–9.
2. Boyer KM, Gadzala CA, Kelly PD, et al. Selective intrapartum chemoprophylaxis of neonatal group B streptococcal early-onset disease. III. Interruption of mother-to-infant transmission. *J Infect Dis*. 1983 Nov;148(5):810–6.
3. Boyer KM, Gadzala CA, Burd LI, et al. Selective intrapartum chemoprophylaxis of neonatal group B streptococcal early-onset disease. I. Epidemiologic rationale. *J Infect Dis*. 1983 Nov;148(5):795–801.
4. Boyer KM, Gadzala CA, Kelly PD, et al. Selective intrapartum chemoprophylaxis of neonatal group B streptococcal early-onset disease. II. Predictive value of prenatal cultures. *J Infect Dis*. 1983 Nov;148(5):802–9.
5. Gotoff SP. Chemoprophylaxis of early onset Group B streptococcal disease. *Pediatr Infect Dis*. 1984 Sep-Oct;3(5):401–3.
6. Puopolo KM, Benitz WE, Zaoutis TE. Management of neonates born at ≥35 0/7 weeks' gestation with suspected or proven early onset bacterial sepsis. *Pediatrics*. 2018;142(6):e20182894.
7. Schrag SJ, Farley MM, Petit S, et al. Epidemiology of invasive early-onset neonatal sepsis, 2005 to 2014. *Pediatrics*. 2016;138(6):e20162013.
8. Ohlsson A, Shah VS. Intrapartum antibiotics for known maternal Group B streptococcal colonization. *Cochrane Database Syst Rev*. 2014;(6):CD007467.

9. Committee on Obstetric Practice, the American College of Obstetricians and Gynecologists. Prevention of Group B streptococcal early-onset disease in newborns. *Obstetrics & Gynecology.* 2020;135(2):e51–e72.

10. Neonatal Early-Onset Sepsis Calculator, Kaiser Permanente Research. https://neonatalsepsiscalculator.kaiserpermanente.org/

11. Achten NB, Klingenberg C, Benitz WE. Association of use of the neonatal early-onset sepsis calculator with reduction in antibiotic therapy and safety: a systematic review and meta-analysis. *JAMA Pediatr.* 2019;173(11):1032–1040.

Reduction of Maternal–Infant Transmission of Human Immunodeficiency Virus Type 1 With Zidovudine Treatment

ANTON H. VAN KAAM AND WES ONLAND

"We found that administering zidovudine to the mother during pregnancy and during labor and delivery and giving it to the infant for the first 6 weeks of life reduced the risk of maternal–infant transmission by approximately two-thirds."

—CONNOR ET AL.[1]

Research Question: In pregnant women with mildly symptomatic human immunodeficiency virus type 1 (HIV), does an antepartum, intrapartum, and neonatal treatment regimen with zidovudine, compared with a placebo, reduce the risk of maternal–infant HIV transmission.

Why Was This Study Done: HIV was discovered approximately 10 years prior to this trial, but it was uncertain how to prevent maternal–infant transmission of this deadly disease, which occurred in 15 to 40% of births with maternal HIV. However, most maternal–infant transmission was known to be in either late pregnancy, during labor, or during delivery.

Year Study Began: 1991

Year Study Published: 1994

Study Location: United States, France (59 centers total)

Who Was Studied: Pregnant women between 14 and 34 weeks' gestation with mildly symptomatic HIV (defined as CD4+ T cell counts >200, who were too well to have indication for antiretroviral therapy, and meeting prespecified laboratory criteria) and their infants.

Who Was Excluded: Pregnant women with ultrasonographic findings for life-threatening fetal anomalies or anomalies that might impact fetal pharmacodynamics or pharmacokinetics of zidovudine, oligo- or polyhydramnios, fetal hydrops, ascites, or anemia. Women who had received any antiretroviral treatment during pregnancy and those who received immunotherapy, anti-HIV vaccines, cytolytic chemotherapeutic agents, or radiation therapy.

How Many Patients: Enrollment was stopped early for improved primary outcome in the intervention group after the first planned interim analysis. The target sample size was 636 mother–infant dyads, and this paper reports the results from the date of the data cutoff for this interim analysis (December 1993). This interim analysis includes 409 mother–infant dyads, but only 363 infants had at least one HIV culture at the time allowing analysis.

Study Overview: This was a parallel-group, masked RCT (Figure 47.1).

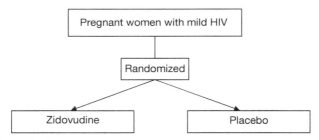

Figure 47.1 Study Overview

What Were the Interventions:
- Mothers randomized to the zidovudine group received a treatment regimen of 100 mg zidovudine orally 5 times daily, which was converted to 2 mg per kilogram body weight (mg/kg) given intravenously for 1 hour at the start of labor, followed by 1 mg/kg per hour until delivery. Infants of these mothers were started on zidovudine after birth, with a dose of 2 mg/kg orally every 6 hours for a total duration of 6 weeks.

- Mother–infant dyads randomized to the placebo group received a placebo treatment not further described in the paper.

How Long Was Follow-up: Up to 18 months for infants; 6 months postpartum for mothers.

What Were the Endpoints:
Primary outcome: Infant HIV infection (any single positive test of 11 tests up to 18 months, as defined by culture of peripheral blood mononuclear cells).
Secondary outcomes: Maternal health status and adverse effects; fetal or neonatal deaths, structural abnormalities, anthropometric measurements, adverse experiences.

Concerns for Bias: The study was at unclear risk for bias in the context of early termination of enrollment, although this followed planned interim analysis. Additionally, the risks for allocation and reporting biases are unclear, as details of random sequence generation, allocation concealment, and predefined outcomes are not provided.

RESULTS

- Zidovudine reduced the risk of maternal–infant HIV transmission (RR 0.68, 95% confidence interval [CI] 0.41 to 0.82, $p = 0.00006$).
- There were no differences between the groups in maternal safety outcomes.
- Infants treated with zidovudine had lower hemoglobin levels during the first 6 months of life, but this difference was no longer present at 18 months. No differences in other neonatal safety outcomes were observed between the groups.

Criticisms and Limitations: It is important to acknowledge that stopping a trial early may lead to an overestimation of the true treatment effect.[2] This knowledge should also be applied to the results of this trial.

Assessment of the primary outcome was hampered as data on HIV status was not available at the time of the interim analysis in 46 (11%) of the included mother–infant pairs. Reassuringly, an addendum from the authors states that data on HIV culture became available for an additional 37 infants and this did not change the findings of the study. Furthermore, in a large proportion of infants, HIV cultures were not available at all follow-up time points, especially after 24 weeks of life. Late positive HIV cultures, especially in the zidovudine group, may have been missed.

Finally, the results of this study are only applicable to HIV-positive mothers with mildly symptomatic disease and without prior treatment with antiretroviral drugs. In contrast, many women in the current era have very low viral loads and are on multiple antiretroviral medications. The results may also differ in HIV-positive mothers with more progressed HIV disease.

Other Relevant Studies and Information:
- Timely activation of research and public health apparatus led the way for this trial's proof of pre-exposure prophylaxis, only approximately 10 years after the discovery of HIV as an "untreatable" new retrovirus.
- Following this study, another 4 RCTs investigated the efficacy and safety of zidovudine in preventing maternal–infant HIV transmission. A meta-analysis of these trials showed a 43% reduction in maternal–infant transmission.[3]
- Secondary analysis revealed increased risk for treatment failure with high maternal weight and conditions associated with fetal exposure to maternal blood or cervicovaginal secretions.[4]
- This treatment continues to be used globally to prevent maternal–infant HIV transmission, now, over 25 years after this study's publication.

Summary and Implications: This study showed that administering zidovudine to mildly symptomatic HIV-positive pregnant women during pregnancy and labor, and for 6 weeks to their infants, reduced the risk of maternal–infant transmission by approximately two-thirds. As a result of this pivotal study, antiretroviral treatment of HIV-positive pregnant women to reduce the risk of maternal–infant transmission became the standard of care. Since the start of prevention of mother-to-child transmission programs, 1.2 million deaths and 2.5 million HIV infections have been averted among children.[5]

A FEW WORDS FROM THE EDITORS

This was one of the first studies that came to mind when planning this book, as it is difficult to imagine a newborn trial with a more profound global impact. This international trial was both admirable and unprecedented in perinatal clinical research at the time, and the collaboration led to the adoption of a life-saving treatment that saved millions worldwide. Like all studies in this book, the impact of even an intervention proven to be efficacious is dependent on the context of care. In high-income

*countries, mothers are now routinely tested for HIV and antiretroviral therapy
would be started as soon as possible. However, a wide range of barriers remain that
negatively impact the uptake in pregnant women, including fear, stigma, and social
exclusion, as well as structural issues in healthcare systems, particularly in resource-
limited settings.[1] Addressing these issues will allow us to more fully access the benefits
proven by Connor et al. back in 1994.*

—Susanne Hay & Roger Soll

1. Razzaq A, Raynes-Greenow C, Alam A. Barriers to uptaking HIV testing among pregnant
women attending antenatal clinics in low- and middle-income countries: a systematic review
of qualitative findings. *Aust N Z J Obstet Gynaecol.* 2021 Dec;61(6):817–29. doi: 10.1111/
ajo.13430.

References

1. Connor EM, Sperling RS, Gelber R, et al. Reduction of maternal-infant transmission of human immunodeficiency virus type 1 with zidovudine treatment. Pediatric
   AIDS Clinical Trials Group Protocol 076 Study Group. *New Engl J Medicine.*
   1994;331(18):1173–80.
2. Bassler D, Briel M, Montori VM, et al. Stopping randomized trials early for benefit
   and estimation of treatment effects: systematic review and meta-regression analysis.
   JAMA. 2010;303(12):1180–87.
3. Suksomboon N, Poolsup N, Ket-aim S. Systematic review of the efficacy of antiretroviral therapies for reducing the risk of mother-to-child transmission of HIV infection.
   J Clin Pharm Ther. 2007;32(3):293–311.
4. Shapiro DE, Sperling RS, Mandelbrot L, et al. Risk factors for perinatal human immunodeficiency virus transmission in patients receiving zidovudine prophylaxis.
   Pediatric AIDS Clinical Trials Group protocol 076 Study Group. *Obstet Gynecol.*
   1999;94(6):897–908.
5. UNICEF. Elimination of mother-to-child transmission. UNAIDS 2021 Estimates.
   https://data.unicef.org/topic/hivaids/emtct/

48

A Randomized Controlled Trial of Magnesium Sulfate for the Prevention of Cerebral Palsy

The BEAM Trial

ELIZABETH FOGLIA

"Magnesium sulfate may reduce the chance that cerebral palsy will subsequently be diagnosed in a child who was a high risk for preterm birth."
—ROUSE ET AL.[1]

Research Question: Among women at imminent risk of preterm delivery between 24 and 31 weeks' gestation, does administration of magnesium sulfate, compared with placebo, reduce the risk of stillbirth or infant death at one year or moderate/severe cerebral palsy among surviving newborns at or beyond 2 years of age?

Why Was This Study Done: Magnesium sulfate was hypothesized to be protective against cerebral palsy (CP) for its role in reducing vascular instability and mitigating hypoxic and other damage.[2] Prior to this trial, 2 large trials each reported a nonsignificant reduction in the composite outcome of death or cerebral palsy following antenatal magnesium sulfate therapy in similar populations.[3,4] However, published evidence from these RCTs was unavailable when this study was launched.

Year Study Began: 1997

Year Study Published: 2008

Study Location: United States (20 centers)

Who Was Studied: Pregnant women at risk of imminent delivery between 24 and 31 weeks' gestation and their infants.

Who Was Excluded: Women with: anticipated delivery within 2 hours or cervical dilation exceeding 8 cm, rupture of membranes <22 weeks' gestation, hypertension or preeclampsia, contraindications to magnesium sulfate, receipt of magnesium sulfate within 12 hours, or major fetal anomalies.

How Many Patients: 2241 women (2336 infants were included in the primary outcome)

Study Overview: The BEAM (Beneficial Effects of Antenatal Magnesium Sulfate) trial was a parallel-group, masked, RCT (Figure 48.1). Randomization was stratified by gestational age (<28 weeks and ≥28 weeks).

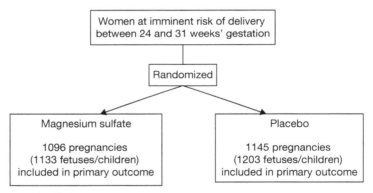

Figure 48.1 Study Overview

What Were the Interventions:
- Women randomized to the magnesium sulfate group received intravenous magnesium sulfate therapy (6 g bolus followed by infusion of 2 g/hour).
- Women randomized to the placebo group received an identical-appearing placebo.

How Long Was Follow-up: 2 years

What Were the Endpoints:
Primary outcome: Composite outcome of stillbirth or infant death by one year CA or moderate or severe cerebral palsy (CP) at or beyond 2 years of CA.
Selected secondary outcomes: CP alone, maternal outcomes and complications, adverse events potentially attributable to the study intervention.
Note, unit of analysis was the pregnancy.

Concerns Regarding Bias: The study was at overall low risk of bias.

RESULTS

- No difference in the composite primary outcome of infant death or moderate/severe CP was detected between patients in the magnesium group (11.3%) and placebo group (11.7%) (RR 0.97, 95% CI 0.77 to 1.23, $p = 0.80$).
- Moderate or severe CP was less frequent in the magnesium sulfate group (1.9% versus 3.5%; RR 0.55, 95% CI 0.32 to 0.95).
- Death was reported in 9.5% of the magnesium sulfate group and 8.1% of the control group (RR 1.12, 95% CI 0.85 to 1.47).
- Adverse events were more frequent among women treated with magnesium sulfate (77.3% versus 12.4%; $p < 0.001$), but no life-threatening events or maternal deaths occurred in either group.

Criticisms and Limitations: It is worth noting that 419 of 2241 (18.7%) maternal participants (18.3% of the magnesium group, 19.0% of the control group) were exposed to magnesium sulfate before randomization, as previous treatment for tocolysis was not an exclusion criterion, if outside of the 12 hours preceding enrollment. Subgroup analyses demonstrated no significant differences in safety or efficacy outcomes based on previous magnesium sulfate exposure, although these analyses may have been underpowered.

Observed rates of moderate or severe CP among survivors in the control group (3.5%) were lower than anticipated (8%). The authors speculate this difference may have resulted from their rigorous methodology to diagnose CP. Because the composite outcome was largely driven by mortality rates, the lower-than-expected CP event rate reduced statistical power to detect a difference in the primary outcome.

Generalizability may be limited for the following reasons: First, over half the women (58%) assessed for eligibility did not meet inclusion criteria. Among those who did, the most common eligibility criterion for enrollment was premature rupture of membranes. Consequently, most enrolled women (97.2%) were able to receive antenatal corticosteroids. Lastly the trial enrolled patients from 1997 to 2004, and thus did not include patients at risk of preterm delivery at the contemporary limits of viability (22 to 23 weeks' gestation).

Other Relevant Studies and Information:

- Two large concurrent trials each reported a nonsignificant reduction in the composite outcome of death or cerebral palsy following antenatal magnesium sulfate therapy in similar populations.[3,4]
- A subsequent 2009 Cochrane systematic review and meta-analysis of 5 trials (including this trial; 6145 infants total) favored magnesium sulfate therapy to reduce the risk of CP among children born to women at risk of preterm birth (RR 0.68, 95% CI 0.54 to 0.87).[5] The number of women needed to treat for benefit to prevent one case of cerebral palsy was 63 (95% CI 43 to 155).
- Soon thereafter, multiple professional societies endorsed or recommended magnesium sulfate therapy for neuroprotection before anticipated early preterm birth.[6-8]
- Magnesium sulfate therapy was not associated with improvement at school age.[9]

Summary and Implications: The BEAM trial demonstrated magnesium sulfate to be a safe and effective intervention to prevent moderate or severe CP among children born to women with threatened preterm birth. Magnesium sulfate therapy is now the standard of care for this indication.

A FEW WORDS FROM THE EDITOR

The impact of magnesium sulfate for neuroprotection of the preterm fetus could be called uncertain. The Cochrane meta-analysis, in which the BEAM trial is included, suggests that we have a broad estimate of the number of infants needed to treat to prevent one case of cerebral palsy, ranging from as few as 43 to as many as 155 fetuses. Importantly, when followed to school age, these infants demonstrated no differences in neurological, cognitive, behavioral, growth, or functional outcomes. Nonetheless, multiple professional societies rushed to endorse the use of magnesium sulfate therapy for neuroprotection before anticipated early preterm birth. Why? Perhaps because, if believed, magnesium sulfate represents a low-cost solution to one of the most consequential problems suffered by preterm infants. Despite these recommendations, many fewer women at risk of preterm delivery are treated with magnesium sulfate compared with the widespread adoption of antenatal corticosteroids, perhaps reflecting the uncertainty regarding the impact of these results on practice.[1]

—Roger Soll

1. Wolf HT, Huusom L, Weber T, et al.; EPICE Research Group. Use of magnesium sulfate before 32 weeks of gestation: a European population-based cohort study. *BMJ Open.* 2017;7(1):e013952.

References

1. Rouse DJ, Hirtz DG, Thom E, et al. A randomized, controlled trial of magnesium sulfate for the prevention of cerebral palsy. *N Engl J Med.* 2008;359(9):895–905.
2. Hirtz DG, Nelson KN. Magnesium sulfate and cerebral palsy in premature infants. *Curr Opin Pediatr.* 1998;10:131–7.
3. Crowther CA, Hiller JE, Doyle LW, et al.; Australasian Collaborative Trial of Magnesium Sulphate (ACTOMg SO4) Collaborative Group. Effect of magnesium sulfate given for neuroprotection before preterm birth: a randomized controlled trial. *JAMA.* 2003;290(20):2669–76.
4. Marret S, Marpeau L, Follet-Bouhamed C, et al. [Effect of magnesium sulphate on mortality and neurologic morbidity of the very-preterm newborn (of less than 33 weeks) with two-year neurological outcome: results of the prospective PREMAG trial]. *Gynecol Obstet Fertil.* 2008;36(3):278–88.
5. Doyle LW, Crowther CA, Middleton P, et al. Magnesium sulphate for women at risk of preterm birth for neuroprotection of the fetus. *Cochrane Database Syst Rev.* 2009;(1):CD004661.
6. American College of Obstetricians and Gynecologists. Magnesium sulfate before anticipated preterm birth for neuroprotection. Committee Opinion No. 455. *Obstet Gynecol.* 2010;115:669–71.
7. The Antenatal Magnesium Sulphate for Neuroprotection Guideline Development Panel. *Antenatal Magnesium Sulphate Prior to Preterm Birth for Neuroprotection of the Fetus, Infant and Child: National Clinical Practice Guidelines.* Adelaide: The Australian Research Centre for Health of Women and Babies, The University of Adelaide; 2010.
8. Magee L, Sawchuck D, Synnes A, et al. Magnesium sulphate for fetal neuroprotection. *J Obstet Gynaecol Can.* 2011;33(5):516–29.
9. Doyle LW, Anderson PJ, Haslam R, et al.; Australasian Collaborative Trial of Magnesium Sulphate Study G. School-age outcomes of very preterm infants after antenatal treatment with magnesium sulfate vs placebo. *JAMA.* 2014;312:1105–13.

Health Services

49

Newborn-Care Training and Perinatal Mortality in Developing Countries

The First Breath Study

DANIELLE E. Y. EHRET

"Essential Newborn Care training and implementation was not associated with a decrease in the primary outcome of neonatal mortality. In secondary analyses, implementation of this program was associated with a significant decrease in stillbirths but not with a decrease in perinatal mortality."

—CARLO ET AL.[1]

Research Question: Does training birth attendants in the World Health Organization (WHO) Essential Newborn Care (ENC) course or the addition of a modified version of the American Academy of Pediatrics Neonatal Resuscitation Program (NRP) reduce the rate of death from all causes in the first 7 days after birth (early neonatal mortality), as compared with standard care, among infants with birth weights ≥1500 g born in rural communities in developing countries?

Why Was This Study Done: Prior to this study, limited observational studies suggested that the WHO ENC course improved midwives' knowledge and skill and reduced early neonatal mortality rates among low-risk women who delivered in first-level clinics in Zambia.[1-3] The First Breath study broadened the educational effort to all delivery room staff and to various birthing settings.

Year Study Began: 2005

Year Study Published: 2010

Study Location: Argentina, Democratic Republic of Congo, Guatemala, India, Pakistan, Zambia

Who Was Studied: All births ≥1500 g (measured or estimated), including stillbirths

Who Was Excluded: Births <1500 g

How Many Patients: The ENC intervention was assessed among 57,643 infants from 96 communities; the NRP intervention was assessed among 62,366 infants from 88 communities.

Study Overview: The First Breath Study included 2 sequential community-based interventions. The ENC intervention was assessed using a before-and-after design (Figure 49.1). Subsequently, the NRP intervention was assessed as a parallel-group, unmasked, cluster-randomized, controlled trial (Figure 49.2).

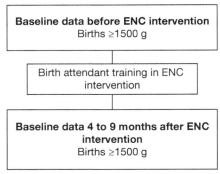

Figure 49.1 Study Overview, ENC intervention.

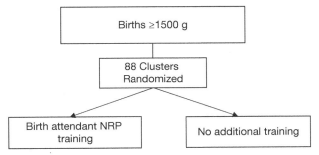

Figure 49.2 Study Overview, NRP intervention.

What Were the Interventions: The interventions were 2 sequential community-based training programs, the WHO ENC course, and a modified version of NRP. All clusters received training in ENC, and 88 of 96 were subsequently randomized (by site of practice) to either training in a modified version of NRP or no additional training.

- The ENC intervention consisted of birth attendant training in routine neonatal care—defined as initiation of breathing and resuscitation (including bag-and-mask ventilation), thermoregulation, early and exclusive breastfeeding, skin-to-skin care, care of small babies, recognition of danger signs, and recognition and initial management of complications (including differentiating stillbirth and early neonatal death).
- The NRP intervention consisted of birth attendant training with in-depth, hands-on training in basic knowledge and skills of resuscitation. This included initial steps in resuscitation and bag-and-mask ventilation; but did not include training in chest compressions, endotracheal intubation, or administration of medications.

How Long Was Follow-up: 7 days

What Were the Endpoints:
Primary outcome: Death from all causes within 7 days (early neonatal mortality rate).
Selected secondary outcomes: Death attributed to birth asphyxia, stillbirth, neurologic outcome.

Concerns Regarding Bias: The first phase (the ENC study) was not a RCT and therefore at inherent risk for confounding,[4] although known important confounding domains were appropriately addressed. As they were unmasked, both the ENC and NRP studies were at high risk of bias due to misclassification of stillbirth and live birth followed by neonatal death, and unbalanced misclassification between groups.[4,5]

RESULTS

- In the initial ENC training phase, there was no significant reduction in early neonatal mortality rate with ENC training (RR 0.99, 95% CI 0.81 to 1.22), and no reduction in perinatal mortality rate (RR 0.85, 95% CI 0.70 to 1.02). There was, however, a significant reduction in the rate of stillbirth from 23.0 per 1000 to 15.9 per 1000 (RR 0.69, 95% CI 0.54 to 0.88, p <0.01).
- In the cluster-randomized trial of a modified version of NRP, training did not reduce the rates of early neonatal mortality, stillbirth, or perinatal mortality.

Criticisms and Limitations: Mortality typically is an objective outcome. However, inherent in the definitions of neonatal mortality rate or early neonatal mortality rates is the denominator of "per 1,000 live births." A limitation in the design of this study is the high risk of bias in the measurement of this primary outcome, as the risk of misclassification of live birth and stillbirth changes with neonatal resuscitation education, which is included in both ENC and NRP interventions. Before ENC training, a liveborn infant who was pale or cyanotic, apneic, and limp may have been misclassified as a stillbirth and put aside without intervention. This infant's classification by ENC-NRP definitions would be liveborn; neonatal death without intervention. Neonatal resuscitation changes the method or algorithm of diagnosis of "fresh stillbirth," from initial visual inspection to a diagnosis of exclusion, made only after an infant fails to respond to neonatal resuscitation efforts taught in ENC and NRP. This risk of classification bias must be considered when interpreting the stillbirth and neonatal mortality rates as reported in this study.

The other major criticism of this study is the lack of implementation metrics for the 2 complex and comprehensive educational training packages. With education as the intervention, several gaps remain in our understanding of the necessary trajectory from intervention to impact. To assess the fidelity of the educational intervention and training cascade, we must more fully understand the acquisition, application, and retention of knowledge and skills and the system of care in which they are applied, including barriers and facilitators to appropriate use. These contextual and implementation factors allow a richer assessment of effectiveness, which can inform assessments of generalizability.

Other Relevant Studies and Information:
- The results and lessons learned from this study helped to inform the development of Helping Babies Breathe, an evidenced-based neonatal resuscitation training program developed specifically for resource-limited environments.[6]

Summary and Implications: The First Breath Study showed that training rural community-based birth attendants in 6 developing countries in the WHO ENC course was not associated with a reduction in early neonatal mortality or perinatal mortality rates, although the rate of stillbirths was reduced. Subsequent training in NRP did not significantly reduce the mortality rates. This study highlighted the misclassification issue of stillbirths, and underscored the importance of understanding, measuring, and improving both stillbirths and neonatal deaths. This trial has led to practice change, and an evolution in neonatal resuscitation education.

A CONVERSATION WITH THE TRIALIST: WALDEMAR CARLO

Given the success of Essential Newborn Care (ENC) training with midwives in Zambia, can you add any insight into the lack of effect of the ENC phase of this study? What about considerations regarding the addition of NRP training in the later phase of this study?

There were important differences between the Zambia and First Breath trials that explain the differences in effectiveness of ENC. The Zambia ENC Trial was a hospital-based trial in which resuscitation training had been implemented in all facilities before ENC was introduced. Thus, fresh stillbirths were not decreased but early neonatal deaths were substantially decreased.

The First Breath Trial was conducted in communities where various levels of health care providers were trained. The ENC component of this trial resulted in a significant reduction of stillbirths. This study was designed as intention-to-treat, so the investigators challenged themselves to reach every single delivery. 19% of the deliveries were assisted by family members and non-trained providers. However, in the 81% of the deliveries in which the intervention was used (ENC-trained birth attendant), there was a significant reduction in perinatal deaths. The large reduction in stillbirths may have prevented a reduction in neonatal mortality.

Have you observed further impact of your trial interventions after the conclusion of this trial?

This was a real-world large-scale implementation of a simplified neonatal resuscitation program whose contents were used to develop Helping Babies Breathe.

... There have been about a million fewer stillbirths and neonatal deaths per year and a steep decline after a few years of this publication. . . . I am sure stillbirths and neonatal deaths will continue to be decreased by these interventions.

References

1. Carlo WA, Goudar SS, Jehan I, et al. Newborn-care training and perinatal mortality in developing countries. *N Engl J Med.* 2010;362(7):614–23.
2. McClure EM, Carlo WA, Wright LL, et al. Evaluation of the educational impact of the WHO Essential Newborn Care course in Zambia. *Acta Paediatr.* 2007;96(8):1135–38.
3. Chomba E, McClure EM, Wright LL, et al. Effect of WHO newborn care training on neonatal mortality by education. *Ambul Pediatr.* 2008;8(5):300–304.
4. Sterne JA, Hernán MA, Reeves BC, et al. ROBINS-I: a tool for assessing risk of bias in non-randomised studies of interventions. *BMJ.* Published online October 12, 2016:i4919.
5. Sterne JAC, Savović J, Page MJ, et al. RoB 2: a revised tool for assessing risk of bias in randomised trials. *BMJ.* 2019;366:l4898.
6. Niermeyer S, Little GA, Singhal N, et al. A short history of Helping Babies Breathe: why and how, then and now. *Pediatrics.* 2020;146(Supplement_2):S101–S111.

50

Effectiveness of Family Integrated Care in Neonatal Intensive Care Units on Infant and Parent Outcomes

EVANGELIA MYTTARAKI AND CHRISTOPHER GALE

"Family Integrated Care improved infant weight gain, decreased parent stress and anxiety, and increased high-frequency exclusive breastmilk feeding at discharge, which together suggest that Family Integrated Care is an important advancement in neonatal care."
—O'BRIEN ET AL.[1]

Research Question: Among infants admitted to the NICU and their parents, does Family Integrated Care (FICare), as compared to standard care, improve infant and parent outcomes, safety, and resource use during hospitalization?

Why Was This Study Done: NICU parents experience anxiety, stress, and a sense of loss of control; and potential benefit to both infants and parents from parental involvement in care had been suggested. FICare was one of the first pragmatic approaches to enable parents to become primary caregivers in the NICU.

Year Study Began: 2013

Year Study Published: 2018

Study Location: Canada, Australia, New Zealand (26 centers total)

Who Was Studied: Infants ≤33 weeks' gestation with no or low-level (e.g., non-invasive) respiratory support and their parents.

Who Was Excluded: Infants who received palliative care, had a major life-threatening congenital anomaly, were on high-level respiratory support, were thought unlikely to survive, or were born to parents unable to participate because of health, social, or language barriers.

How Many Patients: 26 centers were randomized, and one FICare center withdrew prior to analysis. 25 centers (involving 1,786 infants and their parents) were included in the intention-to-treat analysis.

Study Overview: This trial was a parallel-group, cluster-randomized controlled trial; randomization was at the level of the NICU (Figure 50.1).

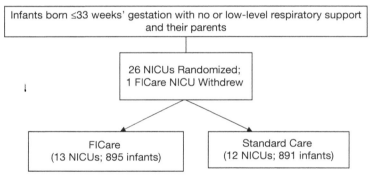

Figure 50.1 Study Overview

What Were the Interventions:

- In NICUs randomized to FICare, parents were integrated into the care of their infants. Such parents consented to spend up to 6 hours a day with their infant in the NICU; attend special education sessions; participate in daily medical rounds; undertake basic infant charting; and provide care for infants with nursing supervision in the areas of feeding, bathing, dressing, and holding skin to skin. These parents were also provided with a program of psychosocial support and other assistance through informal peer-to-peer support and veteran parent and social work involvement in education sessions.
- In NICUs randomized to standard care, routine bedside NICU care was provided by nurses.

How Long Was Follow-up: Hospital discharge

What Were the Endpoints:
Primary outcome: Infant weight gain at 21 days (measured as change in weight Z-score).
Selected secondary outcomes: Weight gain velocity, high-frequency breastfeeding at hospital discharge (defined as ≥6 breastfeeds/day), parent stress and anxiety, infant mortality, and major neonatal morbidities.

Concerns Regarding Bias: This study was at high risk for bias in several aspects. Selection bias may have been introduced, as only parents enrolled at FICare sites were required to commit to extensive involvement in the NICU. This may explain why some parent and infant characteristics differed between FICare and standard care arms.
There was risk for performance/ascertainment bias, as providers were not blinded to the intervention. In addition, due to differential policies regarding transfer, there were discordant proportions of available data for feeding status at discharge (60% FICare versus 89% standard care), leaving these outcomes at risk for attrition bias.

RESULTS

- There were differences in key demographic factors between FICare and standard care groups. Notably, the FICare group was comprised of more infants 22 to 28 weeks' gestation (50% versus 42%) and more Caucasian mothers (74% versus 67%).
- Infants in the FICare group had a smaller reduction in weight Z-score at day 21 (–0.071 [standard deviation 0.42] versus –0.155 [0.42]; p <0.0002).
- The average daily weight gain was slightly higher among infants in the FICare group, as was the rate of high-frequency breastmilk feeds.
- Parental stress and anxiety scores were lower in the FICare group.
- There were no significant differences between groups with regard to mortality, major morbidity, duration of oxygen therapy, and duration of hospital stay.

Criticisms and Limitations: This large, international cluster-randomized controlled trial was a considerable achievement that overcame many of the obstacles associated with this trial methodology. There are, however, limitations inherent in this study which must be considered. Families enrolled in FICare centers were distinctly different from families enrolled at standard care centers. Only families who were willing to make a serious commitment to bedside care were able to enroll at FICare centers, leading to meaningful differences between the 2 populations being compared.[2] It is difficult to know how much these preexisting differences may have influenced the study outcomes independently of FICare, but for some outcomes (such as measures of parental stress and anxiety, and breastfeeding measures) this may have been considerable.

Important differences in feeding status at discharge are hard to interpret, given the different transfer practices between centers.

The primary outcome selected in this trial, weight gain at 21 days, may not be one of the most important outcomes to parents or healthcare professionals.[3] The clinical significance of this outcome, how it relates to long-term measures of child development, nutritional status, cognition and wellbeing, is unclear.

Other Relevant Studies and Information:
- Subsequent evaluations of this cohort suggested FICare may be effective at reducing maternal stress and anxiety[4] and improving later behavioral outcomes.[5]
- Another small cluster-randomized trial in Canada reported reduced length of hospitalization with a similar approach to care.[6]
- Challenges of FICare implementation include change of culture, staff engagement, a change in professional roles, patient safety, legal responsibility of care, lack of parental facilities, communication issues, and institutional barriers.[7]

Summary and Implications: NICU care interrupts bonding between infants and parents, which is detrimental to both parties. FICare recognizes the importance of infant–parental bonding, placing the "care-by-parent" model in the center. This international, multicenter, cluster-randomized controlled trial was unique in examining the benefits and harms of FICare through the gold-standard methodology of a randomized comparison. The cluster design was challenging to implement and led to biases that must be considered when interpreting the trial. However, this trial provides the most robust data to support the benefits of parental involvement in NICU care.

A CONVERSATION WITH THE TRIALIST: KAREL O'BRIEN

Was it difficult finding units that would agree to implement all of the Family Integrated Care (FICare) arm requirements?

In Canada almost all the CNN sites agreed to participate in the trial. The sites that did not had concerns re the trial design rather that the requirements of the study. All sites had to agree to be randomized to FICare or control except Mount Sinai Hospital (MSH) which had completed the pilot study.

The implementation teams from the intervention sites were invited to Toronto for a 2-day training workshop to help prepare them for their local implementation. After FICare was implemented the study implementation team from MSH did an in-person assessment at each site (including an interview of parents, nurses, and physicians) to ensure that all sites were meeting all the requirements of the study and data collection procedures. We also virtually participated in their site steering committee meetings to assist with problem solving around any challenges with implementation.

References

1. O'Brien K, Robson K, Bracht M, et al. Effectiveness of Family Integrated Care in neonatal intensive care units on infant and parent outcomes: a multicentre, multinational, cluster-randomised controlled trial. *Lancet Child Adolesc Health*. 2018;2(4):245–54.

2. Gale C. Family Integrated Care for very preterm infants: evidence for a practice that seems self-evident? *Lancet Child Adolesc Health*. 2018 Apr;2(4):230–231.

3. Webbe JWH, Duffy JMN, Afonso E, et al. Core outcomes in neonatology: development of a core outcome set for neonatal research. *Arch Dis Child Fetal Neonatal Ed*. 2020;105:425–31.

4. Cheng C, Franck LS, Ye XY, et al. Evaluating the effect of Family Integrated Care on maternal stress and anxiety in neonatal intensive care units. *J Reprod Infant Psychol*. 2021;39(2):166–79.

5. Church PT, Grunau RE, Mirea L, et al. Family Integrated Care (FICare): positive impact on behavioural outcomes at 18 months. *Early Hum Dev*. 2020;151:105196.

6. Benzies KM, Aziz K, Shah V, et al. Effectiveness of Alberta Family Integrated Care on infant length of stay in level II neonatal intensive care units: a cluster randomized controlled trial. *BMC Pediatr*. 2020;20(1):535.

7. Patel N, Ballantyne A, Bowker G, et al.; Helping Us Grow Group (HUGG). Family Integrated Care: changing the culture in the neonatal unit. *Arch Dis Child*. 2018;103:415–19.

INDEX